BYE-BYE BABYFAT

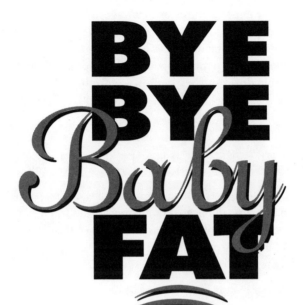

BYE BYE Baby FAT

Reshaping the

new mother...

mind and body

SANDRA TREXLER ED.D.
MICHAEL TREXLER PH.D.

THE SUMMIT GROUP • FORT WORTH, TEXAS

This book is not intended to be a substitute for professional medical advice. The reader should regularly consult a physician regarding any matter concerning her health, especially in regard to any symptoms that might require diagnosis or medical attention. Medical science is an ever-changing field. Every effort was made to insure that the medical information contained in this book was the most accurate and current at the time of publication. Any mention in this book of actual products sold does not constitute an endorsement by the publisher or the authors, except where noted.

THE SUMMIT GROUP
1227 West Magnolia, Suite 500, Fort Worth, Texas 76104

Printed in the United States of America

10   9   8   7   6   5   4   3   2   1

Library of Congress Cataloging-in-Publication Data

Trexler, Sandra, 1961-
    Bye bye baby fat: reshaping the new mother, mind and body
/ Sandra Trexler, Michael Trexler.
        p.cm.
    Includes bibliographical references and index.
    ISBN 1-56530-131-5: $24.95
    1. Postnatal care. 2. Puerperium. 3. Reducing. 4. Physical fitness for women. I. Trexler, Michael, 1952-. II. Title. III. Title: Bye-bye baby fat.
RG801.T74 1994
613'.04244—dc20   94-8918
                                                      CIP

Cover design by David Sims
Pagination by Sean Walker

TABLE OF CONTENTS

PART ONE

YOUR BABY IS HERE; NOW WHAT?

PART TWO
BODY CONTOURING PRINCIPLES

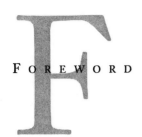

FOREWORD

*a*s a mother two times over, I am intimately familiar with the roller coaster ride known as the "postpartum period." Although I had read literally volumes of books on pregnancy and childbirth to prepare myself for this wonderful adventure, I was on my own once my babies arrived. There was no manual for how to survive the months following a Cesarean section and sleepless nights with colicky babies.

I certainly wish *Bye-Bye Babyfat* had been around when I was pregnant with Lauren and Hannah. In this book, Sandy and Mike have done an excellent job helping new parents understand and embrace the mystery of the postpartum period. In both a professional and personal manner, they provide a practical guide to getting your body and life back into shape after childbirth. With this guide, young couples have a helpful companion as they enter the truly exciting stage of life called parenthood.

Here's a book to add to your library on childbirth and child rearing. Baby isn't the only needy creature in your home. If you take care of Mom, too, everyone's life is a lot more enjoyable!

—Peggy Wehmeyer
ABC-TV news correspondent and mother of two

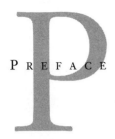

PREFACE

Why this book was written:

Finally! It was my turn. I began to feel the contractions that indicated both a beginning and an end were in sight. A beginning of new life, Michael Linn Trexler, Jr., a beautiful, healthy, perfect baby boy. And an end to the oversized body I had been lugging around for several months—or so I thought.

Throughout pregnancy I had envisioned that all of my excess weight would disappear with the birth of my baby. I gained forty pounds and was convinced that it was "all baby." It wasn't. I will never forget the shock of stepping on the scales the day after giving birth, and discovering that I still weighed almost twenty pounds more than when I first became pregnant. To make matters worse, I seemed to lose my "starlike" status as the bearer of new life, and baby Michael became the focus of everyone's attention.

People couldn't say enough about how beautiful he was and how healthy he looked. His little eight-pound, six-ounce body was flawless. Mine on the other hand, the body that had sacrificed for nine months to help make him that way, was sagging, pain-ridden, overworked, and overweight. Standing in front of my hospital mirror, I still looked six months pregnant, only now I didn't get all the positive attention that comes with actually being six months pregnant.

I read every book I could get my hands on while I was pregnant. There were books which discussed what to expect, what to do, what to eat, how to exercise, and what to avoid to maximize my baby's potential. Not only that, I also was seeing my doctor regularly, even weekly for the last month, and was always prepared with a long list of questions. Information was plentiful and I absorbed it.

But as my delivery day approached, my interests changed. Suddenly, I became concerned about what would happen to me after my baby was born. Many of my pregnant friends expressed similar concerns. Where were we to turn for information about the postpartum period? There would be no more doctor visits, except for one postpartum checkup at six weeks. The pregnancy books did not discuss in detail how, when, or if I would get my figure back. And what about my health? After delivery, my body was aching and it was painful to sit up in bed. I wondered how or if I could possibly feel well again.

Ninety-one percent of pregnant women, like me, reportedly consider regaining their figures as a top concern during pregnancy, along with a few other appearance and health issues. A wealth of information exists in the pregnancy books regarding Kegal exercises and pelvic tilts, and that information is important for regaining muscle tone and function. But no one ever lost an ounce of fat doing these types of calisthenics.

What was missing from the pregnancy book shelves was a comprehensive guide to take women, step by step, through a program that helps them lose body fat, tone and contour muscles, and maximize their health and appearance after having a baby.

The *Bye-Bye Babyfat* program is designed to do all those things. It utilizes the same principles that went into developing a healthy baby, and it works. We all want the best for our babies and will stop at nothing to insure they have the opportunity for perfect development. This book was developed for those of you who want to put the same kind of effort into becoming the healthiest and most attractive that you can be after your baby is born. Optimal health and appearance go hand in hand.

Experts report that 95 percent of all "weight-loss" programs fail. Yet, the weight-loss industry makes billions of dollars making people dependent on their services. Our program is different. We provide you with the information and methods that you can use—on your own—to achieve your health and appearance goals for a lifetime. Compared to carrying a baby for nine months and enduring labor and delivery, following this program is quite simple. Instead of having postpartum depression, you will make a postpartum impression on everyone you see. They will want to know your secret. You will tell them it is commitment and consistency—the same kind that it takes to have a baby.

This book is designed to help you achieve optimal health, while enhancing your physical appearance and body shape, in about three months. Whether you've just had a baby, or have had children years ago and never shaped up, this program will work for you. It is most effective, however, to begin the program as soon as possible after your baby is born. The postpartum period is characterized by a heightened interest in learning and readiness to change by the new mother. In other words, right after having a baby we are open to change and ready to consider new lifestyle habits. We have what researchers call a psychological readiness for learning new skills.

This program offers effective, yet easy to follow guidelines for after your baby is born, and beyond. It empowers you with the tools you need to have a healthy, shapely body from now on—no pills and no gimmicks. It outlines steps for you to take to shape and sculpt your body and to reduce fat. It also helps you adjust to the postpartum period. In the last chapter of this book, a medical advisory board answers the most common questions women encounter during the postpartum stage.

Bye-Bye Babyfat prepares you for what to expect after your baby is born and helps you focus on taking the steps required to regain, or to experience for the first time in your life, optimal health, body shape, and appearance. It helps you adjust to the emotional ups and downs common during the postpartum period, and motivates you to feel great about yourself and the accomplishments you have made. Your self-confidence will be enhanced, and that will make you even stronger and more effective at accomplishing your goals. The side effects of such a well-balanced physical and mental health program include a shapely body, a youthful appearance, and more energy and enthusiasm than you've ever experienced before.

I postponed having a baby for years, fearing that it meant losing my attractiveness, my fitness, and my health. What I found out instead was that having a baby helped me become more attractive, physically fit, healthy, and happy than ever before. It will do the same for you. The key to success is to begin working on yourself soon after your baby is born—with the same determination that you devoted to his or her development. This book will tell you how. It was the "perfect" program for me, and it will be the perfect program for you, too.

—Sandy Trexler

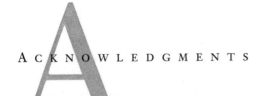

A C K N O W L E D G M E N T S

irst and most importantly, we would like to thank God for His divine guidance and direction in the development and completion of this work. Anything we accomplished is a gift from Him.

Our most special thank-you goes to our son, Michael, who is largely responsible for our inspiration to write this book. We used to worry that having a baby would take us away from our goals. Instead, his arrival has defined them.

We are grateful to our parents, Bill and Betty North, and Lionel and Velma Trexler—thank you for your love, support, and understanding as we focused in on this project. Thanks for always being "there" for us.

A special note of appreciation goes to my mother, who had five babies, and to Mike's mother, who had three—and to all the women who have struggled through the postpartum period with little or no help. Your struggles have helped define our purpose.

We also want to extend a heartfelt thank-you to the following people:

To my brother, Neal, for his encouragement and faithfulness in praying for us daily.

To Uncle Tony, for keeping Michael busy with special "prizes."

To my sisters, Gail, Nancy and Peggy, and to Mike's sister, Vicki, for their support.

To Gary Harrell, for his wisdom; and to Robert Cupp, for his help.

To our community group members, for their concern, especially the Matthews and the Bains.

To Don Bumgarner, for all the many ways in which he has provided support and help.

To E.R. and Poppa Jim, for their love and concern for us, especially for "Mikey."

To Sarah, for the love and attention she has shown Michael during our busiest days.

To Amie, for her help and support.

To the doctors, nurses, and staff at Parkhill Clinic for Women, for seeing the need to provide services to women during the postpartum period, and for allowing me to fill that need in their clinic. A special thanks go to obstetricians George Cole, M.D., Scott Bailey, M.D., James Romine, M.D., David Buckley, M.D., and David Duke, M.D., for contributing their time and insight as our trusted medical advisors. In that regard, thanks also to James Beckman, Jr., M.D., of the Fayetteville Plastic Surgery Clinic, and to Allison Morris, R.N.P., and Kim Moody, M.S., R.D., of the Washington Regional Medical Center for their roles on the advisory board. Also, a heartfelt thank-you goes to Donita Kossover of Parkhill Clinic for her cheerful help in arranging schedules, working out program details, and for her support in general.

To the nurses and staff who have had babies and participated in our programs. We are grateful for their insights and feedback. A special thanks to Sue, Georgina, and René.

To the American College of Obstetricians and Gynecologists. We thank them for the valuable information.

To the many clients and program participants we have had over the years. We thank them for showing us that our program works. Thank you for the feedback.

To Kitty Demars. We thank her for her valued support.

Last, but not least, our most sincere appreciation goes to The Summit Group for catching the vision for this project. Thank you to Mark Hulme, Len Oszustowicz, Dave Gavin, Brent Lockhart, Mike Towle, Liz Bell, Joe Bishop, Walter Kaudelka, and all the others for understanding the need for this book, and for their expertise in making it happen.

INTRODUCTION

ongratulations! You have just opened the pages to what probably is the first weight-loss, health-and-fitness program where you begin with a terrific success—a weight loss of fifteen to twenty pounds with the delivery of your baby. With *Bye-Bye Babyfat*, you also begin a program where you are already in excellent cardiovascular condition, resulting from carrying an extra twenty-five to forty pounds—or more—during the final stages of pregnancy. In other words, pregnancy was great training.

The purpose of the *Bye-Bye Babyfat* program is to help you keep that success going. Many women wait six weeks or longer after delivery before they begin to work on themselves. For healthy women, six weeks is much too long to wait. Being sedentary for six weeks after nine months of carrying a baby causes you to lose most of whatever conditioning you've gained. This slow-down time also allows the extra babyfat you've accumulated during pregnancy to "settle in," and increase. This makes it more difficult to achieve success when you do decide to improve your condition.

On the other hand, an immediate return to activity optimizes and increases the cardiovascular fitness gains you've made during pregnancy, and allows you to work on reducing body fat stores. It also enhances recovery by helping prevent stress incontinence (leaking of urine), a dropping (or prolapse) of the pelvic organs, sexual difficulties, backache, varicose veins, leg cramps, and edema, or bloating.

The type of activity discussed in this book will promote healing of your traumatized uterine, abdominal and pelvic muscles, and will help them regain tone. It will restore the strength and contour of your abdominal and pelvic floor muscles, correct many postural deficiencies which were caused by changes in body shape during pregnancy, and strengthen your chest wall to help support heavy breast tissue. It will contour your body and leave you feeling energized and self-confident.

This program was designed to teach you how to take control of your life and your health in the postpartum period, and how to lose body fat and keep it off for life. So congratulations on making a commitment to your personal well-being. You've taken the first step to becoming the healthiest you've ever been. And congratulations on the success you're about to experience or have already experienced through the birth of your baby.

Remember, nine months of pregnancy is like nine months of training for the Olympics. When you achieve success after nine months of training, don't stop! If an athlete wins a competition and then decides to take six to eight weeks off, she will lose most of the gains she has made. That does not mean she can never get back into peak performance shape, but means that it will take more time and more effort. The same is true for you. Keep the ball rolling while you've already got it in motion.

Your Baby Is Here;

Now What?

Dr. Sandra Trexler

PART ONE

I

Baby's Perfect; You're a Wreck

*I*t was early in the morning, my husband Mike was at work, and I sat down in my upstairs office to write. Everything felt peaceful and under control. This new mom stuff was a piece of cake. For the first time in my life, I didn't even have to get dressed in the morning. I could just stay in my skimpy nightgown until noon. Who would ever know the difference?

Then it happened. A strange smell began to drift through the room. The bottles! I had forgotten about the bottles. (I had put ten new baby bottles and nipples on the stove to sterilize them). As I threw open the office door I stepped into a haze of smoke. The smell of burning rubber and plastic choked me. I ran to the baby's room and grabbed Michael out of his crib. I covered his face, grabbed the portable phone, and ran to the door.

Once outside, I frantically called the non-emergency number to the fire department. A gentleman answered the phone and I explained my situation to him. All I really wanted to know was if it would hurt us to breathe the fumes inside the house. He instructed me not to go back inside until he could send someone to check things out. He assured me this was no big deal and there would be no sirens—just someone to make sure it was safe for us. As I sat on the hood of my car with Michael, I couldn't believe the position I found myself in. Just a few minutes ago everything was under control. Now it was complete chaos.

Off in the distance, the faint sound of sirens grew louder and louder. "Good," I thought, in a morbid kind of way. "Someone else is in worse shape than me." But the sound grew closer. "No! This can't be happening." Around the corner and into my driveway they whipped— one, two, three, four fire engines and an ambulance. Out jumped the first firefighter. How could I tell this man my emergency was burned baby bottles? How could I make my situation sound better, or less *ridiculous? Was this a dream, or was this really happening to me? I used to be in control of my life. It didn't matter. I couldn't even steril- ize baby bottles without creating an emergency scene. But the good news was that everything turned out okay.*

That day was a big part of my introduction into motherhood, and it's been about the same ever since—a series of seemingly insur- mountable obstacles which ultimately turn out to be no big deal. Welcome to motherhood.

The postpartum period is a stressful time for all of us, regardless of our backgrounds. There is no way to be prepared for all the small crises that come with having a baby. However, there are ways to cope more effectively with any situation that arises. It helps to know that we are not alone, and that the emotional ups and downs we experience during the postpartum period are normal. It also helps to be healthy and in great condition. Although it might seem unbe- lievable, this is the optimal time to reshape your body—to make it look and feel better than ever. Indeed, this is an oppor- tunity to make the postpartum period the best time of your life.

An important aspect of effective postpartum adjustment is being prepared for what to expect after delivery. When we are given specific information about what to expect before under- going a painful experience such as an operation or childbirth, we adjust much more quickly and perceive less pain than indi- viduals who were uninformed. Why? Because most of us have a need to feel that we are in control of our lives. Knowing what to expect prepares us. This holds true for that period of time right after our babies are born. Numerous books are dedicated to explaining what to expect from pregnancy and delivery. However, there is little information out there that deals specif- ically with the postpartum period.

One of my postpartum clients, Gloria, expressed a similar concern. "I would open my pregnancy books to sections on stress or postpartum blues, and just wish that I could find more than a small paragraph or two explaining these feelings I was having," Gloria said. "I needed to know I was normal and things would get better. I wanted more specific information. I needed to know other women were feeling like me—that I wasn't the only one. I would just open the same books over and over, hoping I would find more information about postpartum adjustment."

The first step in being able to cope is understanding what you are experiencing and why. You wouldn't think of going into labor and delivery without being informed regarding your participation in the birth of your baby. We believe it's even more important for you to be aware of what you can expect after your baby is born, and to know how to use this time to become the best you can be. (Remember, you have complete control over what happens to you now—much more so than in labor and delivery—but only if you're prepared!)

POSTPARTUM EMOTION

The First Few Days

"MY FIRST FEW DAYS HOME with my newborn baby boy will be filled with excitement and elation," I told myself as I lay in my hospital bed, just after giving birth. I couldn't believe that this precious creature was mine. I felt like I had done such a great job with my pregnancy that surely— more than any Olympic athlete— I deserved a gold medal. Everyone would probably be waiting to tell me what a great job I had done, and my day of glory was finally here. Or was it?

As a new mother, I was shocked by my sudden loss of "star" power. I was no longer on center stage. Everyone kept telling us how beautiful our little baby was: "He looks like who? I guess he does look a little bit like his father." How could people say that when he obviously looked just like me! "Hey, don't forget me," I screamed in my mind. "I'm the one responsible for how he turned out." Did anyone want to hear about the sacrifices I made—about the vitamins I took, or the wine I didn't? Or what about the walks I took and the dessert I didn't?

It was as if Michael had just come out that way, independent of anything I had done. Everyone marveled at Michael. For the first time, this baby I had been carrying around as a part of me for nine months was separate from me. It felt like I had been training for the Olympics for forty weeks and had won the race, only to have a new little star take my place on the podium for the applause and the medal ceremony. I felt left out. Everyone wanted a part of baby Michael. I also felt possessive. He was mine. He was supposed to prefer me, but he really didn't seem to care who was meeting his needs. I wanted to run away to a deserted island with the baby. I felt selfish. I wanted to go back to my doctor every week and hear him say that I was doing perfectly. I wanted to be perfect. I wanted to be thin and to feel sexy. I wanted more energy and less pain. I wanted my family around, but they annoyed me. I wanted another dose of pain medication to ease this rather large dose of reality—things were just not like I had expected.

> *It felt like I had been training for the Olympics for forty weeks and had won the race, only to have a new little star take my place on the podium for the applause and the medal ceremony.*

I worried about keeping my baby healthy. Everyone touched him and breathed on him. My dog, Sami, delivered puppies a couple of weeks before I had Michael. I watched her as people approached the puppies. She growled and snapped at anyone who tried to get near them. She would seem embarrassed after making such a scene, but it was just her instinct. I wasn't much different than Sami. I felt so protective of Michael, even with people I normally would have trusted.

I felt the need to kill every germ that came in contact with the baby. If someone kissed his cheek, I would use an antibacterial wipe on it. (He ended up getting a rash from the wipes!) I wouldn't put the baby in the infant seats provided by shopping centers (germs), and I covered his face when people walked by (to filter out germs). My husband was much less concerned about such things. I worried about everything and disliked worrying, and was angry about my husband's apparent lack of concern. I worried that no one else was worrying enough.

It wasn't until later that I realized what I experienced when I first came home from the hospital were normal postpartum feelings and emotions. These were triggered by changes to which my body and my mind were adjusting, and by the drastic changes in my lifestyle (stress overload!). Not everyone is affected by these changes in the same way, but everyone goes through postpartum adjustments and postpartum stress.

The physical and emotional changes that come with pregnancy are many. Most of these changes occur over a forty-week period. They are gradual. All of these pregnancy changes must be reversed after delivery. The majority of the hormonal readjustments happen rapidly during the early postpartum period—a time which lasts only one-sixth as long as pregnancy—or about six weeks. That period of time can be an emotional roller coaster, and it is briefly mentioned in most pregnancy books. But for most of us, this six-week early adjustment period is just the beginning. Real postpartum stress and adjustment often lasts for months and even years after delivery.

Many of us have been led to believe that the entire process of postpartum adjustment takes place within the first six weeks. When that doesn't happen (and in most cases it won't) we begin to feel abnormal—as if there must be something wrong with us. I was certainly not expecting to feel like I did. I thought it would be a peaceful time to relax and enjoy my baby. And I was certain that if I did experience some stress, it would be gone in six weeks.

Who was the "expert" who came up with the theory that postpartum adjustment lasts only six weeks? Remember, it took nine months of adjustment to complete a successful pregnancy. Doesn't common sense tell us that it would take at least as long and even longer to adjust back to normal? Think of it like this: The pace of adjustment during pregnancy versus the pace of adjustment during postpartum could be compared to running two marathons, twenty-six miles out and twenty-six miles back. Say you are an average marathon runner and can run the course in four hours. At that steady pace your body will experience many ups and downs and overcome many obstacles before you finish the race.

Suppose after finishing, and resting a short time, you must begin the return trip of twenty-six miles. You are already fatigued, certain you gave everything you had to complete the first marathon. As you approach the starting line for the return course, you are told there is one additional requirement. You must travel the twenty-six-mile course back in only forty minutes, or one-sixth as long as it took you to run the course going out. Not only do you have to run back when you are already tired, but you have to return in one-sixth the time. Sound impossible? It is.

> ■ ■ ■ ■ ■ ■ ■
> *P*ostpartum adjustment is a process of adapting to many physical and mental changes, and much like pregnancy, it takes time and effort.

Postpartum adjustment is a process of adapting to many physical and mental changes, and much like pregnancy, it takes time and effort. You have as much of a chance completing postpartum adjustment in six weeks as you do running a marathon in forty minutes. However, you can make great strides during the first six weeks after delivery toward reaching your postpartum goals, and laying a foundation for optimal health and adjustment.

Postpartum adjustment is probably the toughest challenge you will ever face. Think about our marathon example. What if a friend said, "I know an easier, more effective way. Jump in my car and I will drive you back." Would you hitch a ride? Of course you would. We're making a similar offer to you for postpartum adjustment. It is a long and seemingly impossible journey alone, but we know an easier, quicker, and more effective way. Jump in with us and we will help take you where you want to go.

One of the most popular, yet misleading beliefs in modern society is that giving birth and caring for an infant are instantly a fulfilling and rewarding experience. This is rarely the case. In reality, giving birth is a traumatic, life-crisis event. After delivery, many new mothers are afraid. They might feel uncertain of their new roles and responsibilities. Disappointment and concern about their physical condition is commonly reported. From working with postpartum women, and through my personal experience, I have come to realize that this period of life is probably one of the most difficult times women face.

Many women feel they are "abnormal" or "bad" because of postpartum's confusing emotions. They are reluctant to tell their spouses, physicians, or even other women about their feelings. Women tend to feel ashamed when reality doesn't measure up, because they have always expected to feel pure joy.

Because no one is talking about these feelings, we all sit around thinking we're the only one who's abnormal. Postpartum stress can last up to several years after the birth of a baby if a woman has not made all the necessary adjustments, including regaining her physical shape. Postpartum stress is compounded when women do not feel the freedom to share feelings and emotions, or when they feel as if they are abnormal. This stress can be relieved when women learn that they are normal, their feelings are common, they are not alone, and when they learn how to get their lives and their bodies back in shape.

"This group has been an answer to prayer for me," Lisa told me while leaving a Bye-Bye Babyfat group meeting. "It has been so comforting to hear all these women share their personal experiences. I thought I was the only one who felt so strange. I never dreamed other women had the same kinds of thoughts and reactions after having a baby as me, so I never told anyone how I was feeling," she explained. "I thought I must be crazy because I have been so emotional since my baby was born.

"Feeling like I was going crazy made me lose confidence in myself, and I started believing I couldn't be successful at anything—including losing weight. I had practically resigned myself to being fat and unhappy for the rest of my life. When I came to these meetings and started to understand the postpartum experience, I realized I was normal and my confidence began to grow. Now I've learned to manage my stress, to feel great about myself, and I've lost eight pounds in five weeks."

No two women experience the exact same emotions while they adjust to their newborns and to the postpartum period. But there is some common ground for all of us. We all must make major adaptations which are learned. Becoming a mother does not come naturally. Even if you've had babies before, each new infant causes more change and requires new adjustments. Your first emotions toward the baby will probably be excitement, possessiveness, disappointment, ambivalence, or elation. Any of the above would be considered normal.

When we fall in love with our husbands, everyone expects us to go on a honeymoon. We are expected to get away with this person and to spend time just enjoying being alone and discovering everything about them. I wanted a honeymoon with my baby, too, but instead I was expected to share his affections with many other people. To me, it felt like people were vultures hovering around my precious baby, just waiting for an opportunity to snatch him up.

My resentment toward people who desired to be a part of Michael's life grew each day, and so did my feelings of selfishness and guilt. Looking back on the experience, I realize that feeling possessive is natural and is commonly experienced by other women during the early postpartum period. It would have been helpful for me to have been prepared to expect these types of feelings, and to have known they were normal.

Typically, after a baby is delivered, a mother will first experience feelings of exhilaration about the birth. She will be relieved if everything went well. As she approaches the second postpartum day, the excitement fades as she attempts to recover from the discomfort of delivery. By the third day, she might feel tearful and alarmed by a lack of emotion for the child, or she might feel terrific and awed by her baby. Any number of responses could be considered normal. In most cases, feelings of love and closeness toward her infant will develop and grow as the new mom spends more time with the baby.

Think of a major event in your life. It was probably preceded by a buildup of excitement and anticipation, and almost always followed by a letdown. That's just part of life. It's impossible to live and function at peak levels of emotion and enthusiasm all the time, and there must be a time of readjustment and balance. If you are married, you likely remember the "letdown" often experienced by newlyweds after the wedding. I can remember falling in love with my husband and thinking that I had been blessed with the prince of the universe—the perfect man. I was so happy that I didn't need food, or sleep, or any of the other boring necessities of life. I had Mike, and I was living on a cloud!

I'll never forget how disillusioning it was the first time thunder shook my cloud. It was our first argument and I learned that I would have to come back down to earth. My knight in shining armor was not perfect (and neither was I), and we had to go through the storming phase of our relationship.

One of my university professors once explained that with any new relationship there are four dominant phases—forming, storming, norming, and performing. In other words, there is the beautiful coming together phase (forming) when a relationship is formed, followed by a turbulent phase (storming) where positions in the relationship must be defined and individual differences understood. Then comes a normalizing phase which could be compared to a calm after a storm, when things settle down and regular patterns are established, and finally, a performing phase, when it becomes possible to develop the relationship to its highest potential.

I thought of this analogy often during the first few years of my marriage, and again when Michael was born. It seemed to hold true in both relationships. So don't be surprised if you enter a stormy period soon after your baby is born. Knowing that it's temporary and natural can help minimize the negative impact.

EMOTIONAL ADJUSTMENTS
AFTER DELIVERY

FOLLOWING THE BIRTH OF EACH BABY, there is a series of predictable phases that women must work through.[1] Those might include:

- reliving labor and delivery

- grief over the outcome

- concern about your infant's performance

- disappointment about your body's condition

- gaining confidence in mothering skills

- redefining the roles of family members

- making the transition from patient to caregiver

- ambivalence about motherhood

Let's look at each one in a little more detail:

1 Reliving labor and delivery

You want to compare your actual delivery to the expected one—the one you had in mind. These are normal feelings. Reliving and questioning your delivery experience is a common postpartum response. What could you have done better? Why did your doctor insist on giving you medication when you had planned on going natural? Why did he perform an episiotomy when you had requested that he not?

Most of us dream of a perfect, fantasy delivery. If the experience was long and difficult, an unplanned C-section had to be performed, an extensive episiotomy was necessary (as in my case), or any number of complications arise, mothers often

---

[1]R. Mercer, "The Nurse and Maternal Tasks of Early Postpartum," *The American Journal of Maternal Child Nursing* (The American Journal of Nursing Company: New York, September-October 1981) pp. 341-345

feel anger and disappointment. Asking questions of your doctor, nurse, or midwife will help you to better understand why certain actions might have been taken and will help you accept reality.

The actual experience of labor and delivery rarely measures up to the fantasy experience we imagined. That is why it is very important to have a physician or caregiver you trust. In the heat of the moment, he or she might have to make decisions that are different from those you have previously discussed, and the well-being of your baby could depend on those decisions.

> ■ ■ ■ ■ ■ ■
> *The* actual experience of labor and delivery rarely measures up to the fantasy experience we imagined.

Much of your actual labor and delivery might not be within your control. However, it is quite normal for you to need explanations as to what was done and why. My doctor was patient in explaining why I required a large incision and in reassuring me that it would heal completely. I requested not to have an episiotomy, and I ended up needing the most extensive episiotomy that can be performed. I was very upset that things had not gone as I expected, and I needed to understand why.

Most physicians, nurses, and/or other obstetric specialists understand your need to have your questions answered. In all fields of medicine, it has been shown that the patients who recover most quickly are the ones who participate in their own care. It might sound funny, but the annoying, questioning, demanding patients heal more quickly. The bottom line is, be assertive. Don't be afraid to ask, ask, ask!

2 Grief over outcome

In this phase, you will compare your expectations regarding your fantasy baby with the reality. It is hard to believe that we could actually be disappointed when we are presented with our newborns—even if they are perfectly healthy. Some women might not have these feelings. But feeling some letdown when you see your infant is a normal response. You need not feel guilty. You might be surprised about the sex, the size, or the characteristics of the baby. Or he or she might just look unattractive at first.

One of my postpartum patients, Julie, was extremely disappointed when she first saw her baby boy. When I went to see her in the hospital, she said, "He is the homeliest baby I have ever seen!" She didn't want any visitors because she was embarrassed for them to see the baby. He was a nine-pound, four-ounce, healthy baby boy named Steven. The next afternoon Julie called me on the phone and said Steven was simply the most beautiful baby in the world. It is important to understand that when we first see our babies, they have just been through one of the most stressful events they will ever encounter—the birth experience.

In magazines and on television, babies portrayed as newborns are usually several weeks or even months old. They appear plump and beautiful, smiling and responsive. This causes many of us to expect the Gerber baby immediately after delivery. In reality, newborns are more likely to look thin, wrinkled, rashy, and blood-stained. The skin might appear red or bluish and is covered with varying amounts of a cheesy-looking substance called the vernix caseosa. This covering has protected the baby's skin during its immersion in amniotic fluid.

Depending on your delivery experience, the baby's appearance might be temporarily altered even more. I was upset when my baby came out with a cone-shaped head and with scrape marks on both sides of his face. The marks resulted from the use of forceps and were completely gone within a couple of days. But when I first saw him I thought he was scarred for life. His head was elongated because he was large and was forced through a relatively small birth canal.

I expected a well-rounded, pink-faced, perfectly proportioned, bright-eyed baby to pop out of the womb and greet me. It would have been helpful for me to have known in advance how a healthy newborn really looks. If this is your first pregnancy, here is a realistic description of a typical newborn's initial appearance:

- Newborns are usually between eighteen and twenty-two inches long and weigh from five pounds, eight ounces up to about nine pounds. The head is large in comparison with the rest of the body. It will measure about thirteen to fourteen inches in circumference.

- The face might upset you at first, unless you are prepared to see a broad, flat nose with a receding chin and chubby cheeks. Blisters are often present on the upper lip if the baby has been sucking in the womb.

- On the skull are the two most obvious fontanelles (soft spots). One is above the brow, and the other is close to the crown of the head in back. The bones of the skull are separated, rather than fused as they are in adults. This separation allows the bones to slide over each other as the head passes through the narrow birth canal. This mobility also allows for the infant's rapid brain growth. The brain is protected by a tough membrane and by the scalp. The anterior fontanel at the top of the head will close between nine and eighteen months, and the posterior fontanel in back of the head will close by four months.

- The baby's neck appears short and his/her shoulders small and sloping.

- The abdomen seems large and rounded with an umbilical stump which will fall off in about ten days, revealing the baby's navel.

- Breasts are often swollen. This enlargement is caused by exposure to high estrogen levels while in the uterus and is temporary.

- The pelvis and hips are narrow, and the legs will likely be drawn up against the abdomen in the pre-birth position.

- The skin is thin, dry, and transparent, and you might see the baby's veins. The baby might have a white, creamy coating on the skin immediately after birth. Again, this coating is called vernix, and it is a waxy substance which has protected the skin in the uterus.

- Downy hair on parts of the skin is not unusual. Michael's ears were covered with black, downy hair which disappeared shortly after birth.

- A newborn's eyes appear dark blue and might have a blank, starry gaze. The eyelids might be red and swollen from pressure during the delivery. In most hospitals, antibiotic drops are applied to the newborn's eyes. The drops might cause mild, temporary inflammation. When the baby cries, veins on the head swell and throb and you will notice that there are no tears as the tear ducts do not function yet.

- The genitals of both sexes will seem large in comparison with other body parts. This is due to exposure to maternal hormones.

- The amount of hair on a baby's head is variable. Most of this hair will fall out and be replaced. The color and texture of the new hair might be quite different from that of the hair with which the infant was born.

Immediately after delivery, mucus and other amniotic residue are immediately suctioned from the baby's nose and mouth. The baby begins to breathe regularly and you might hear his/her first wail. The navel cord is clamped and cut, and the baby is wrapped in a warm blanket. The baby is given an Apgar rating. The Apgar test was developed in 1952 by Dr. Virginia Apgar, a renowned pediatrician. It is a method of screening the newborn which allows medical personnel to quickly evaluate the baby's condition—at one minute and at five minutes after birth.

This rating is used to assess whether your baby needs extra medical care immediately. *Each* of five signs is rated on a scale of zero to two, with ten being the best possible *total* score. Scores between seven and ten usually indicate that your baby is in good condition. If the baby scores below seven, he or she should be taken to the nursery for observation and care. Apgar measures the following:

- A = appearance or color

- P = pulse or heart rate

- G = grimace or reflex irritability (reaction such as a cough or sneeze when suctioned)

- A = activity or active movement

- R = respiration or breathing

A normal score at one minute after birth is seven or greater. At five minutes after birth, nine or ten is considered normal.

The newborn's first stool is called meconium, and it might appear black and tarry. Newborns might cough, sneeze, yawn and hiccup. These responses are all normal. He or she also has many reflex responses, such as the startle reflex, grasp reflex, rooting reflex, crawling reflex and walking reflex. You might want to have your pediatrician do an exam at your bedside to show you how your baby responds to certain stimuli.

3 Concern about your infant's performance

This emotional phase comes about as you compare your baby's behaviors to those of other infants, or stories you've heard about other infants. How your infant eats, cries, and burps as compared to others might become your indicators of his or her wellness. Try to realize that all newborns are individuals and will behave differently.

At first, I called the pediatrician if Michael cried too much, or didn't cry enough. I remember one specific time when I called my pediatrician because Michael seemed too sleepy. The doctor's response to me was that I should rejoice, and let Michael sleep. (My husband has teased me about that incident many times, by picking up the phone and saying, "Doctor, my baby is sleepy!")

Your pediatrician should be patient in explaining what you can expect from your baby, and you will want to take advantage of his visit during your hospital stay. The pediatrician will briefly explain how to care for your infant and will ask you if you have any questions. Then you probably will not see him or her again until the baby's two week checkup. Do not hesitate to ask questions about caring for the baby, breast-feeding, or any other concern you might have. Most hospitals have a lactation specialist or a nurse who will help you with breast-feeding. Take advantage of these services before you leave the hospital.

4 Disappointment about your body's condition

As you begin to reconcile your expectations about your fantasy baby with reality, you must also accept the reality of your postpartum body. You might still look six months pregnant. You will likely step on the scales only to find your weight still lingering twenty pounds or more above your pre-pregnancy weight. This was one of the most difficult times for me. I had not expected to be left with so much excess weight after delivery. Immediately after her baby is born, the mother is usually only about twelve pounds lighter. The baby accounts for about seven to nine pounds, the placenta one to two pounds, and the amniotic fluid and lost blood another one to two pounds.

Many women are disillusioned to discover that they still appear pregnant after delivery.

Many women are disillusioned to discover that they still appear pregnant after delivery. Within the first week, the mother will typically drop another five pounds of fluid through urination. Much of the remaining excess weight is probably fat tissue and must be eliminated carefully through a structured activity and nutrition program. Using our Body Contouring Program, I was able to regain my pre-pregnancy size and shape quickly. So can you! Within six weeks of delivery, you could be wearing your pre-pregnancy jeans. You might wish to go beyond that and achieve the shape you've only dreamed of before. We will discuss some feelings and emotions about your postpartum body later in this chapter.

Gaining confidence in mothering skills

It is helpful to allow some room for learning, and not to expect perfection at first. If you have never played tennis, you wouldn't expect to walk out on a court and be able to automatically know how to hit beautiful shots and win a match, simply because someone handed you a racquet. In a similar way, you can't be expected to automatically know the skills involved in handling and caring for an infant, without the help of others. Utilize the knowledge and expertise of nurses, pediatricians, family, and friends, and don't feel guilty for not knowing everything about mothering. It's probably a myth that women have a complete set of inborn mothering skills. You experienced moms know what I'm talking about.

Redefining roles of family members

It is often difficult to incorporate the changes brought about by the new baby into your former routine. Therefore, everyone in the family has to make adjustments. Patience and understanding on the part of each family member is helpful as you adjust to a new addition. (Chapter 11 was written specifically to help men understand what their wives are going through physically and emotionally, how to help them adjust, and how to adjust themselves during the postpartum period.)

7 Making the transition from patient to caregiver

This involves the transition from the dependent role of patient to the busy and complex life that awaits you at home.

This transition is sudden and abrupt, and is especially difficult for many women. I have found that almost all new moms need to develop new, more effective coping mechanisms after childbirth. Some of the most important coping strategies you can use are discussed in the stress management section of this book.

Sometimes, the reality of sharing your life with an infant is overwhelming—although you love the baby more than you ever

■ ■ ■ ■ ■ ■ ■ ■ ■

*T*he home often becomes the sight of chaos and leaves you with the sense of being out of control.

thought you could love anyone. The home often becomes the sight of chaos and leaves you with the sense of being out of control. Again, feeling out of control is stressful. In addition, the focus has changed from when you were pregnant. During pregnancy, everyone is concerned about your needs and your well-being. You are the "patient"—the recipient of everyone's care and concern. Once the baby is born and you leave the hospital, you become the caregiver and the baby is the patient—the focus of everyone's attention and concern.

8 Ambivalence about motherhood

There might be times when you experience ambivalent feelings about motherhood and you might feel trapped. You might also feel jealous as the attention of others shifts from concern for your well-being to concern for the baby. Feelings of abandonment are common, as well-meaning friends and relatives overwhelm the baby with attention, and ignore you. Feelings of jealousy might also arise between you and your spouse, as you both spend increasing amounts of time focused on the baby. The relationship between mates, and between you and your baby's siblings, is stressful during this period of readjustment to changing roles.

Even if you are adjusting to these problems quite well, the postpartum period is a time of change and adaptation, which means it is a time of stress for everyone in the family—especially you! You might need more understanding and more information. As stated before, think of yourself as an athlete in training. Most athletes need a coach to help them become their very best. This book will be your coach as you become your postpartum best!

Although most of us have prepared for labor and delivery throughout pregnancy, the transition into the role of mother is rapid and difficult.[2] Too often we are not prepared in advance for what to expect beyond delivery. Disappointed expectations cause a great amount of stress. Simply knowing that what you are experiencing and feeling is "normal" will help you in making the transition.

Remember that asking questions and requesting assistance will help you regain control of your life in the first few postpartum days. This is a time for learning and patience. Emotional feelings of warmth and attachment toward the baby will evolve and your confidence as a mother will grow. Getting yourself together will help you better care for the baby, improve your energy level, enhance your confidence, and help you cope. We believe the postpartum period is the perfect time for a lifestyle improvement.

[2]M.A. Auvenshire and M.G. Enriquez, *Comprehensive Maternity Nursing: Perinatal and Women's Health.* 2d edition. (Jones and Bartlett: Boston, Massachusetts, 1990)

CHAPTER TWO

Medically Speaking: The First Two Weeks

I believe I'll go through labor much more easily than other women," I announced somewhat arrogantly to my husband on the way to the hospital.

"Is that so?" he responded with an air of doubt which angered me.

"Absolutely!" I replied. "I'm used to pain. I've been working out for years. I have developed a very high pain tolerance. That's why I don't believe I'll need any medication. Most women just have not conditioned themselves to tolerate pain the way I have. I'm in such good shape that I should be able to push the baby out quickly," I explained. I was so confident. I was so naive! I was so wrong!

Looking back now, I think of my eighteen hours of labor as one of my most humbling life experiences. Contractions transformed me from a powerful, strong-minded, athletic woman determined to have a simple, controlled, drug-free delivery—to a whining wimp who would have welcomed just about any drug I could possibly get.

"Would you like some Demerol to take the edge off those contractions?" the nurse asked.

"Will it be okay for the baby?" I asked.

"It will be fine for the baby," she said.

"Then yes, I'll take as much as you'll give me," I replied. And it was done. Even though labor did not turn out like I had planned, I still had delivery. That's when I would show my true colors. I would really shine in delivery.

"Push!" the nurse said as she pressed hard on the top of my abdomen. "Sandy, we need you to push."

"I'm trying, but I can't feel anything," I explained. And I really couldn't feel anything. I thought I was pushing, but I really couldn't even tell. The doctor was explaining that things were taking a little longer because the baby's head was being blocked due to the shape and size of my tailbone. I just lay there, wondering if my labor would ever end, and tried to push when I was told to.

Things seemed to drag on and on with no progress. I could hear some snipping noises, but I couldn't see much of anything. Then, suddenly, the doctor's voice rang out, and he said with excitement, "Here's the head!" All I could see was the expression on my husband's face. He was awe-inspired. And now it was here—the moment we had been anticipating for so long.

"It's a boy, it's a big boy," the doctor announced.

I looked down and was consumed by the miracle—this little person, the one who had grown inside my body for the previous nine months, was now here in the same room with us. At that moment, I had feelings of joy and accomplishment that I had never experienced before, and have not since. One of my professors had described her delivery experience to me early in my pregnancy. I remembered her words. She said, "Sandy, when my son was born and the doctor held up this perfect little baby boy, I felt such overwhelming joy that I said, 'Lord, if this is all there is—if there is nothing more in life for me than this moment—it's enough!'"

I understood exactly what she meant. It was the most indescribable feeling of completeness I've ever known, or even dreamed possible.

It seemed like an eternity passed and I was still lying on the table waiting for the doctor to finish doing whatever he was doing. The nurse explained that the doctor had to repair a little damage. (It was actually a lot of damage from my fourth-degree episiotomy that I still didn't even know I had). Finally, one hour after Michael's delivery, the doctor was finished and I was able to really hold my son (while I was being sewn up, I was in an awkward position and couldn't hold him the way I wanted to.)

The baby nursed instantly, my family came in and saw him, and everything was wonderful. A little while later I was taken to a private room and a nurse came in to check on us. She explained to me that I needed to call her for pain medication immediately when I began to feel a hint of pain, because with an "episiotomy like you had," I would need to keep the pain controlled. "What are you talking about?" I asked.

"He didn't tell you?" she replied. "The doctor was forced to *perform an extensive episiotomy for Michael's delivery—a fourth-degree episiotomy." I should have realized what was going on, but I didn't. "What is a fourth-degree episiotomy?" I was familiar with the word episiotomy, but this "fourth-degree" stuff was new to me. I had not read much about episiotomies, because I was not planning on having one.*

*F*ew women have deliveries which measure up to their expectations, although we go through so much education and preparation regarding what we should do during our labor and delivery. For many of us, very little of this experience ends up being within our control. There are a few lucky ones who go through it without a hitch. The rest of us must accept some modifications. If you've already delivered, it might be helpful to understand exactly what was done and why. If you will be delivering soon, it is wise to understand all of the possibilities, and not to be completely set on one type of delivery.

There is one primary goal for labor and delivery—to bring your baby into the world in the healthiest way possible. For some of us, achieving that goal means things might not go as we planned. That's why it's so important to have a doctor or midwife that you trust completely. It also is helpful to remain flexible and open to change, just in case an alternate delivery method is necessary. Remember, the primary goal is to have a healthy baby—the method of delivery soon fades into a distant memory.

HOW WAS YOUR DELIVERY? ■

THERE ARE SEVERAL DIFFERENT WAYS for a baby to enter into the world. Therefore, it is helpful to understand the type of delivery you had, and what you can do afterward to facilitate recovery.

Vaginal delivery is the most common type. But not all

vaginal deliveries are the same. A woman may have a natural vaginal delivery where no medication is taken, or she may choose to use medication for pain relief. She may have a vaginal delivery in which her perineum (area between the vagina and rectum) stretches adequately to allow the baby to pass through, or she may have varying degrees of tearing or incision into the perineum (episiotomy).

In any case, a vaginal birth involves the delivery of the baby through the birth canal and through the vagina. The beginning of delivery is said to take place when the baby's head first appears at the opening of the vagina. Delivery is completed when the baby's feet slip out. As delivery begins, the baby's head no longer slips back between contractions. The mouth of the vagina opens wider and wider, and changes in shape from a slit to an oval to a circle. As the baby's head descends farther, the entire perineum bulges more and more until the vagina begins to open around the baby's head. When the vagina is spread widest by the emerging head, crowning is taking place.

If drugs are not used, crowning is said to cause a painful, burning sensation, which is quickly followed by a tingling or numbness caused by the pressure of the baby's head on the nerves and blood vessels in the area. If medication is given, it is likely that the mother will feel little or no discomfort during delivery, even if she has an episiotomy. Between 70 and 85 percent of babies are delivered vaginally.

Another type of delivery is the cesarean section (C-section). This is when the baby is removed through a surgical incision into the abdomen and into the uterus. About one in four of all deliveries are performed by cesarean section. Several factors might lead doctors to perform a cesarean delivery.

■ One factor is abnormal labor or failure of labor to progress properly. This is called dystocia, the most common cause of cesarean deliveries. The most common type of dystocia, or abnormal labor, is when the mother's pelvis is unable to accommodate the fetal head.

This condition (sometimes called cephalopelvic dispro-portion or CPD) simply means that, for some reason, the baby's head cannot pass through the mother's pelvis for a vaginal delivery. The mother's pelvis might be too small or might be shaped such that it blocks passage of the baby's head.

■ Another factor could be a breech, where babies come out buttocks or feet first.

■ A third factor that might require cesarean is fetal dis-tress, whereby the infant is not tolerating labor well.

With advanced technology, doctors are able to monitor the con-dition of the fetus during labor. They can monitor the baby's heart rate and detect potential problems. Repeat cesareans (doing a C-section with a second baby because a woman had one with the first) are performed in some cases, but less often than they used to be.

A few years ago, medical experts routinely advised that once a woman had a cesarean section, she must have one for all subsequent deliveries. Their concern was that a woman's uterus might rupture where it had been cut before if she tried to have a vaginal delivery. But when doctors began to make cesarean incisions horizontally, instead of vertically, and in the lower part of the uterus, the risk of future rupturing during vaginal deliv-ery was greatly reduced.

There are other less common factors which might lead to a cesarean delivery. One is an abnormal placental attachment. The placenta, which provides nourishment to the fetus, might be attached to the uterus in such a way that it blocks the open-ing of the cervix. This condition, called placenta previa, makes it impossible for the baby to pass through the cervix for a vagi-nal delivery. In some cases, there might be a separation of the placenta from the wall of the uterus (abruptio placentae) which would endanger the baby and make an emergency C-section likely.

There also are cases in which the umbilical cord slips through the cervix and is in danger of being compressed by the baby's head. This could cut off oxygen to the fetus. This is called prolapse of the umbilical cord and usually requires a C-section. Some maternal infections also make cesarean deliveries necessary.

The woman who has a cesarean has undergone surgery as well as childbirth, and she might experience more pain and fatigue. However, early walking is still generally recommended for enhancing recovery. Again, you need to consult your physician and obtain his or her approval. In many cases, after cesarean delivery, you might not feel like you can begin walking for a couple of days. But the sooner you are able to walk the more quickly you will begin to feel better. In most cases, the more you do, the more you can do. However, it is especially important for cesarean patients to remember not to lift anything heavier than the baby until you have been cleared to do so by your doctor.

◼ MEDICATIONS

SEVERAL TYPES OF PAIN-RELIEF MEDICATIONS which might be given to the mother during delivery have minimal side effects on the baby. Demerol is a commonly used obstetrical analgesic (powerful pain reliever). It is often given in low doses during labor to reduce some of the discomfort associated with contractions. Many women (myself included) report that it relaxes them and makes them better able to cope with contractions. Demerol also is often give to the mother to relieve pain during the early postpartum recovery period.

During the late stages of labor, a regional nerve block (anesthetics injected along the path of certain nerves to block pain) might be given. Regional blocks are preferred over general anesthesia because the mother can remain awake during the birth and will be alert afterwards. Several types of blocks are available. A pudendal block (administered through a needle inserted into the perineal or vaginal area) reduces or eliminates pain in the perineal area, but does not relieve uterine or abdominal pain. In other words, a woman will still feel the pain of contractions, but will not feel pain in the vaginal area. The pain-killing effects of a pudendal block can last throughout delivery and the repair of an episiotomy.

To relieve pain of uterine labor contractions and the pain associated with delivery, two basic types of regional anesthesia are commonly used: epidural blocks and spinal blocks. An epidural block (anesthesia is injected outside the dural space, not in the spinal fluid) stops most feeling below the waist, yet allows the mother to move her legs and to help push. It can be given continuously during the latter part of labor. Epidurals are commonly used for both vaginal and cesarean deliveries. They are popular because a relatively small amount of drug is needed to relieve pain. Epidurals are administered by a small tube that is inserted through a needle into the epidural space outside the dural sac containing the spinal fluid and spinal cord.

■ ■ ■ ■ ■ ■

Regional blocks are preferred over general anesthesia because the mother can remain awake during the birth and will be alert afterwards.

A less frequently used form of epidural anesthesia is the caudal block. It is inserted lower down the back than a lumbar epidural, can be given with the patient lying on her side, and it might require more medication to be effective.

A spinal block (a single shot of anesthesia injected into the spinal fluid, between the lumbar vertebrae in the lower part of the spine) also stops most all feeling below the waist; however, it removes the mother's ability to push. In such a case, the baby must be delivered with forceps or a vacuum extractor, or by cesarean. It is given very late in labor because the effects might not last long. A low spinal or saddle block is often used for forceps-assisted vaginal deliveries.

EPISIOTOMY ■

SOMETIMES A SURGICAL INCISION in the perineum is necessary to facilitate vaginal delivery. This incision is called an episiotomy.

It is usually about two inches long and is made from the bottom of the vagina downward toward the anus, or slightly to one side. If the incision is made straight down the midline of the perineum (from the bottom of the vagina toward the top of the anus) it is called a midline episiotomy. This type of incision is the simplest type of episiotomy to repair. Because the incision is made along the natural line of the tissue, this type of episiotomy heals well and results in less blood loss than a mediolateral incision (discussed below). However, the major disadvantage of the midline episiotomy is the possibility that it will be extended down through the anal sphincter as the baby's head is delivered. Doctors performing midline episiotomies must be skilled at repairing the anal sphincter and the rectal mucosa should the incision be expanded.

An incision which is angled off to one side is called a mediolateral episiotomy. This type of incision begins at the bottom of the vagina and is cut at a thirty-degree angle from the midline of the perineum. Because it cuts across the tissue, it is less easily repaired and more susceptible to complications of healing than a midline incision. There is also more bleeding and more pain with a mediolateral episiotomy. The advantage to this type is that it is less likely to extend into the anal sphincter. Both types of episiotomies are repaired after delivery of the placenta and after the cervix and the vagina have been examined for lacerations (tears).

Lacerations or episiotomies might extend to the vagina and cervix, around the urethra, into the uterus, and to the perineum. They are graded by degree according to the amount of tissue that is involved. A first-degree incision or laceration involves only the skin or mucosa. A second-degree also involves the underlying muscle, as well as the skin and mucosa. A third-degree involves even more tissue, and includes the skin, mucosa, underlying muscle, and the anal sphincter. A fourth-degree is similar to a third, but is further expanded to include the rectal mucosa. This is an important concept to understand, because when the nurse told me I had a fourth-degree episiotomy, I had no idea what she was talking about. Things seemed worse because I didn't understand what was happening to me or why.

Episiotomies became popular in the United States in the 1920s, when the use of forceps became popular. Since 1980, the use of forceps has greatly declined. Yet, it is estimated that 62 percent of all deliveries and 90 percent of all first-time vaginal deliveries are performed using an episiotomy.

Doctors give several reasons for the routine use of episiotomies. Many prefer a controlled episiotomy incision to the possibility of an uncontrolled tear or laceration. In many cases, especially with first-time mothers, the perineum will tear if an episiotomy is not performed. Some doctors believe that by enlarging the vaginal opening, an episiotomy might prevent stretching of the muscles and ligaments around the perineum, thus reducing or minimizing perineal trauma. Preventing such stretching would also prevent other problems, including weakening of the muscles which support the bladder, uterus, and rectum. That means a woman would be less likely to experience such troubling conditions as a fallen uterus, protruding rectum, and urinary leakage.

Some argue in favor of episiotomies, stating that they shorten the second stage of labor by as much as thirty minutes. This reduces the amount of pressure to the fetal head by decreasing the time the baby's head is pushing against the pelvic floor. In many cases (such as my own delivery), an episiotomy is not an option, but a necessity. An episiotomy might be the most desirable option, if the mother has an unusually muscular perineum that does not stretch easily (common among athletic women), or if the baby presents in a difficult position, if the baby is very large, or if it is so small that its skull is fragile.

Episiotomies are usually required when one or more of the following conditions exist:

■ rapid labor, with no time for perineal stretching

■ uncontrolled delivery

■ abnormal presentation of the baby

■ large baby, rigid perineal tissue and instrumental deliveries (use of forceps, vacuum extractors, etc.)

The incision is typically made between contractions, and local anesthesia is almost always given. Repair of the incision usually takes about fifteen to thirty minutes (longer in some cases). While there is some discomfort in the healing of the episiotomy, it is not reported to be significantly greater that the perineal discomfort associated with a vaginal delivery without an episiotomy (unless the episiotomy is a third- or fourth-degree). To relieve discomfort and swelling from perineal wounds, an ice pack is applied immediately after the repair is completed. Ice is used for up to twenty-four hours. After twenty-four hours, a warm sitz bath (soaking in water) is given three or four times a day, and helps relieve pain, cleanse the area, and promote healing through increased circulation. Vaginal and perineal wounds heal quickly due to an abundant blood supply to the area.

■ FORCEPS AND VACUUM EXTRACTORS

EVERYONE HAS HEARD A HORROR STORY regarding the use of forceps. Forceps are believed to have been used since the late 1500s, and there probably have been many instances of serious damage. Before cesarean sections were practiced, forceps were the only option for babies stuck in the birth canal. In modern times, the practice of high forceps, or reaching up high into the mother's pelvis with forceps (probably the practice responsible for the horror stories we hear) is never done. Instead, doctors do a C-section. In some cases, mid, low and outlet forceps are still used.

Mid forceps are used when complications arise and the baby has descended to the level of the mid-pelvis, and engagement of the fetal head has taken place. When forceps are used after the baby's head is down on the perineum, the technique is called low or outlet forceps. These types of forceps techniques, when practiced by a skilled physician, pose no more risk to mother and baby than a C-section.

The vacuum extractor, an instrument which is often used instead of forceps, suctions the infant out of the birth canal using a metal or plastic cup applied to the fetal head. Advantages of using the vacuum extractor are that it does not require as much space as the insertion of forceps, and it is not as likely as forceps to injure or tear the mother's perineum.

CHAPTER THREE

Speeding up Your Recovery

a woman who delivers vaginally with no episiotomy, or with a first- or second-degree incision, usually heals relatively quickly. Any major discomfort is typically gone within one week, and early walking is encouraged (within eight to twelve hours). A woman who delivers vaginally with a third- or fourth-degree episiotomy might experience some discomfort for between ten days and one month after delivery. In most cases, however, it is still beneficial for her to be up walking, slowly and gradually, from the first day after delivery. Five-minute walks, two or three times daily, encourage circulation and promote healing.

It is important for women to consult with their physicians while still in the hospital, and to follow his or her recommendations for early walking. Obtain your doctor's approval to follow the Pre-Conditioning Program we have provided at the end of chapter 5. The walking that you do early provides a foundation for increased activity and optimal healing later.

Listening and paying close attention to your own body is very important. Let's be honest. Any movement you do in the early hours after delivery is going to be a little bit painful. Even lying in bed is painful. However, if you experience any sharp, unusual pain, it could be your body's way of saying something is not right. Any time you experience such pain while walking, stop and consult your physician.

It is also important for you not to do any heavy lifting. You should avoid lifting anything heavier than your baby for the first two weeks after delivery. If you follow our Pre-Conditioning Program and work up to thirty minutes of continuous walking within two weeks after delivery, you will have prepared your body to lose fat and regain tone in the quickest and safest possible manner.

PHYSIOLOGICAL CHANGES AFTER DELIVERY

Involution of the Uterus

AFTER DELIVERY OF ANY KIND, there are many physiological (physical) changes which take place. The first change begins immediately after delivery of the placenta (the baby's life-support system while in the uterus), and is referred to as the involution of the uterus. This change involves a shrinking of the uterus back to pre-pregnancy size. During pregnancy, the uterus has grown to about fifteen times its normal size in order to accommodate the growing baby.

In the first hour after delivery, it is critical for the uterus to remain firmly contracted. Muscle fibers in the uterus must contract in order to clamp off dilated blood vessels. If it were to relax, the woman could lose a large amount of blood. The uterus also must contract in order to begin shrinking back to its original size.

Due to pregnancy, the uterus has risen to the level of the navel, and it remains there for about the first twenty-four hours after delivery. It weighs about one thousand grams (a little over two pounds). Periodically, the nurse might apply pressure or massage the uterus to stimulate contraction. This type of massage might help express any blood clots and help prevent the uterus from becoming relaxed.

Massage of the uterus might be mildly painful for those who have delivered vaginally, and can be very painful for those who have delivered cesarean—yet it is necessary. Beginning on the second postpartum day, the uterus descends about one centimeter below the navel each day. The ligaments that hold the uterus in place do not regain tone as quickly as the uterus itself. Therefore, the uterus might seem loose and is easily moved about in the abdomen the first few postpartum days. By the end of the first postpartum week, the weight of the uterus is decreased by half, to about five hundred grams. At six weeks, the uterus weighs only about sixty grams (three ounces).

Shedding of the Uterus Lining

THE ENDOMETRIAL LINING (inner lining) of the uterus separates into two layers during the first three days postpartum. The upper layer is sloughed off or shedded in the form of a vaginal discharge called lochia, and the lower layer becomes the basis of the new endometrium. The lochia discharge progresses through three stages:

- First you will notice a bloody discharge (rubra lochia) which is red, has the odor of fresh blood, and continues to flow for one to three days. This discharge contains blood and mucus.

- Next, the discharge will fade to a brownish color (called serosa lochia) and indicates that healing of the placental site is taking place. It is thicker and lighter in color than rubra, and lasts up to ten days.

- Finally, you will experience a white discharge (alba lochia) which sometimes lasts until six weeks after delivery.

Any abnormal discharge should be reported to your physician. This would include such things as a steady flow of bloody discharge (rubra) with no decrease or with frequent soaking of perineal (sanitary) pads, any foul odors, or any other symptom that seems out of the ordinary.

After vaginal delivery, the cervix is relaxed and very congested with blood. It might have several lacerations of various sizes due to the trauma of birth. In only eighteen hours, it will have regained much of its pre-labor form and by the seventh day, the cervix is dilated only about one centimeter.

Vaginal Shrinking

DELIVERY STRETCHES THE VAGINA, which is often left bruised, swollen, and stretched out so much that it might gape open for a couple of days. During the next few weeks, the vagina will shrink down a great deal. To restore muscle tone of the muscles surrounding the vagina (which aid in sexual pleasure and in bladder control) perform the postpartum exercises described in the Pre-Conditioning Program.

Hypothermic Reactions

Many women experience uncontrollable shaking in the early postpartum period (first forty-eight hours after delivery). This chilling or hypothermic reaction usually lasts about fifteen minutes and is often frightening for the new mother. The exact cause of the chilling is not known, but several possible explanations have been offered. It could be caused by:

- the sudden release of intra-abdominal pressure after delivery

- nervousness and exhaustion related to the stress of childbirth

- the side effects of extreme muscular exertion during delivery

- sensitivity to elements of fetal blood (developed during pregnancy)

Development of Hemorrhoids

PREGNANCY OFTEN CAUSES or worsens hemorrhoids as the enlarging uterus puts pressure on the perineal veins. Many women might also have problems with constipation during pregnancy. Labor and delivery compound the problem due to extreme straining. During the first few days after delivery, stool softeners might be given along with Metamucil or some other type of dietary fiber. Increased amounts of liquids also tend to reduce the severity of constipation. If constipation persists, the nurse will probably recomend a laxative. In many cases, walking helps stimulate bowel movements without straining.

Anesthetic sprays and ointments, witch hazel pads (Tucks), and sitz baths all might be used to provide relief of hemorrhoids and general perineal pain. The symptoms associated with hemorrhoids are usually diminished within three weeks after delivery.

Hematomas

DAMAGE TO UNDERLYING BLOOD VESSELS can happen during delivery even without injury to the skin or mucosa. This type of damage could be the result of pressure from the fetal head, pressure from forceps if they are used, or the puncture of a vessel during the insertion of anesthesia. The blood loss from this type of injury might be gradual and a great deal of blood might be lost before the hematoma is found. The most common locations of hematomas are the vulva, the vagina, and the subperitoneal space. Hematomas are suspected if you experience intense pain in the perineal area or notice a discolored bluish or reddish mass.

Bladder Trauma

TRAUMA CAN OCCUR to the bladder or urethra due to the passage of the fetal head through the birth canal, and this can cause tenderness and edema (swelling). Symptoms are even stronger if a woman has a rapid delivery, extended periods of pushing, a forceps delivery, or episiotomy and/or laceration. This trauma might lead to nerve damage which decreases bladder tone. This places a woman at risk for a distended (overfilled) bladder. In other words, your bladder might not be sensitive enough to signal you to empty it before it becomes too full. It might be necessary for the nurse to insert a catheter (instrument inserted internally) to keep the bladder empty for forty-eight to seventy-two hours until the bladder can regain its tone.

Elimination of Excess Fluid

ABOUT TWO TO THREE LITERS of excess fluid was retained during pregnancy. The body begins to excrete this fluid during the first twenty-four to forty-eight hours after delivery. This excretion might be in the form of urine or excessive perspiration. A woman should not be alarmed if she awakens with a soaked nightgown and wet bed linens due to perspiration.

Afterpains

DURING THE FIRST FEW DAYS AFTER DELIVERY, a woman might experience afterpains, or periodic contractions of the uterus. These contractions, which might feel like menstrual cramps, help keep the uterus firmly contracted, and often increase in intensity with each delivery—as the uterus becomes more distended. Contractions might be more intense during breast-feeding. Afterpains are often alleviated by activity, and rarely last more than a few days. If they are extremely painful, consult your doctor.

Engorgement

WHEN THE BREASTS BECOME VERY FIRM AND FULL (they feel as hard as a rock and as though they might explode), the condition is called engorgement. It usually happens for the first time about forty-eight to seventy-two hours after delivery. After the first time, engorgement can happen any time a mother goes too long between nursings. Engorgement is caused by a combination of the filling of the breasts with milk and edema or swelling of the breast tissue. Hot, moist towels or a hot shower help stimulate letdown and milk flow. If the nipple area is extremely firm, the mother might have to express milk until the area is soft enough for the infant to take hold. Nursing will relieve engorgement symptoms. If you are not breast-feeding, check with your doctor for instructions on how to relieve engorgement symptons.

Sore Nipples

UNTIL YOUR NIPPLES HAVE ADJUSTED TO NURSING, they might become sore, red and even cracked. Over time they will toughen up, but until they do, you might want to apply lanolin, which you can get from your pharmacy, to protect nipples. It is also helpful to allow nipples to air dry after nursing. Always allow your nipples to dry before you cover them with a bra. Switch baby from one breast to the other after about five to seven minutes of nursing on one side, for the first few days, so that one nipple doesn't become too sore.

Musculoskeletal System

PROGRESSIVE LORDOSIS (an increasingly larger curve in the lower back) is common for most women as pregnancy progresses. As a woman's abdomen protrudes further and further out during pregnancy, her lower back attempts to compensate and adjust by shifting forward as well. There is also an increased ability of the joints to move due to hormonal changes which allow them to become more flexible. During the last trimester, slumping forward with the shoulders, due to the pulling of heavy breasts, and a forward flexion of the neck also are common. These postural changes can lead to various types of joint pain and lower back discomfort, and need to be readjusted after delivery.

A woman must focus on correcting her posture as she begins to walk in the early postpartum period. It is helpful to concentrate on keeping the shoulders and the head back, and on contracting the abdominal muscles. This helps bring the pelvis into a neutral position (the lower back is straight or flat, not curved forward), removing the exaggerated curve in the lower back.

ABDOMINAL CHANGES

FOLLOWING DELIVERY, the abdominal wall is very loose and overstretched. With a concentrated effort, the abdomen will tighten up in about six weeks. If a woman does not practice abdominal exercises designed to tighten and strengthen these muscles, she will notice a protruding pouch in her abdominal area, and might experience continued lower back pain and other postural problems.

In order to regain abdominal tone, or to achieve it for the first time, you must work at it. It will not happen naturally the way some of the other changes (involution of the uterus) will. As your abdominal muscles become tightened, the loose skin in the area will tighten up as well. You might be left with stretch marks, which will gradually fade but might never disappear completely. But a tight, firm stomach can be achieved!

Sometimes pregnancy might cause the pair of vertical muscles of your abdominal wall to separate. Ask your nurse or doctor to check your abdominal muscles before you do any abdominal exercises to make sure they have not separated. If they have, you should do a special exercise to help them heal. (Do not do any other abdominal exercises until your physician says you are ready.)

To do this special exercise, lie on your back, and cross your hands over your abdomen with your fingers connected in the middle to hold the abdominal muscles together. Exhale as you raise your head slowly, and inhale as you lower it. Do this four or five times, several times daily, until the separation has closed.

The changes we've just discussed are those most commonly reported in the early postpartum period.

Breast is Best

DURING ONE OF OUR WEEKLY BYE-BYE BABYFAT CLASSES, Gail explained that her husband, a very competitive man, was a little jealous when she breast-fed their newborn infant. He was frustrated that she was able to provide something for the baby that he could not. The baby never seemed happy when he was holding her—and it made him feel as if he was lacking in some way.

One evening, Gail was taking a sitz bath and trying to relax in the bathroom. She heard the baby crying and knew she was hungry. But Gail was enjoying her relaxation time, and decided just to let her husband manage the baby for another few minutes. As she sat there, she heard the baby stop crying. Then the baby would cry again and stop, cry and stop. Curious, Gail tiptoed out of the bathroom to see what was happening. As she peered around the corner, she saw her husband, holding the baby to his breast, and attempting to get her to latch on to his breast. The baby would try, but when she couldn't get anything to come out, she would become frustrated and cry.

"I caught him red-handed trying to fake our baby out and make her think that he could breast-feed, too," Gail explained. The moral of this story is that one of the things that makes breast-feeding so special is that it's something only you and your baby can share. There is no way your husband can upstage you in this area.

On a more serious note, experts agree that the ideal food for the newborn baby is mother's milk. The composition of breast milk is quite different from that of cow's milk, and it contains substances which cannot be duplicated in infant formulas. Breast milk contains antibodies against certain diseases, and it has been shown that breast-fed babies are less prone to infections than are bottle-fed babies. Mom's milk also contains T and B lymphocytes (cells known to fight against diseased cells in the body) which could be helpful to the infant's immune system.

For the first five days after delivery, a liquid called colostrum is secreted by the breasts. On or around the fifth day, mature milk begins to flow. Colostrum contains more protein, more minerals, and less sugar and fat than mature milk. Antibodies are present in colostrum, as well as other components believed to increase the infant's resistance to diseases. Mature milk contains proteins, lactose (sugar), water and fat, as well as the immunity factors already discussed.

All vitamins except vitamin K are present in human milk, but in varying degrees. Nursing mothers are encouraged to continue taking prenatal vitamins in order to increase the levels of vitamins in her milk. Since the mother's milk does not contain vitamin K, it is often administered to the infant soon after delivery.[3] Human milk also contains a low amount of iron, although the iron that is present is better absorbed than is the iron from other sources.

---

[3]Norman F. Gant, Paul C. MacDonald, and Jack A. Pritchard, *Williams Obstetrics*. 17th edition (Appleton-Century-Crofts: East Norwalk, Connecticut, 1985)

■ BENEFITS OF BREAST-FEEDING

- ■ Breast milk is more digestible. Therefore, breast-fed babies are less likely to be constipated or to have diarrhea than bottle-fed babies.

- ■ Breast-feeding helps in the development of the baby's mouth structure—its jaws, teeth, and palate—because breast-fed infants must suckle more energetically than bottle-fed infants.

- ■ Breast-fed babies have fewer ear infections and require fewer trips to the pediatrician.

- ■ Breast-feeding helps the mother's uterus contract and return to its prepregnancy size (sometimes you might feel your uterus cramping as you nurse). It might help reduce the flow of lochia more quickly than if you were not breast-feeding.

- ■ Breast-feeding enhances bonding due to the close, skin-to-skin contact required, and it encourages mother/infant time alone. (It is often a good excuse to get time alone with the baby amidst the attention of all the well-meaning friends and relatives.)

- ■ Breast-feeding is less complicated than preparing bottles, and it is far less expensive.

- ■ Breast-fed infants are less likely to become obese than bottle-fed babies.

- ■ There is some indication that breast-feeding reduces the risk of breast cancer in the mother prior to menopause.

Although the benefits of breast-feeding are many, there are some considerations nursing mothers must make. Certain drugs can pass from mother to infant through breast milk. Consult your physician before taking any drug. You must follow the same dietary principles that you adhered to during pregnancy, because as long as you breast-feed, much of what you take into your body is passed on to your baby.

Avoiding alcohol and cigarettes is strongly recommended. Studies show that one glass of wine per day could have an adverse effect on your baby's motor skills development. In large amounts, alcohol can make the baby sleepy and unresponsive.

Many of the toxic chemicals in tobacco enter breast milk and are passed on to the baby. The exact effects of these chemicals on babies is not known, but they are believed to be harmful. Avoid herbal teas, because some herbs are powerful drugs and can affect the baby. Don't eat freshwater fish that could have been contaminated by industrial wastes, and peel and scrub fresh fruits and vegetables before eating to reduce dietary pesticides. Doctors recommend that you limit intake of saccharin products, as well as aspartame (the ingredient in NutraSweet).

Breast-feeding has been said to interfere somewhat with sexual intercourse. The vagina is often dry due to the hormonal changes of lactation. This dryness can be eased by using a vaginal lubricant during intercourse. Nursing mothers should take in at least six to eight ten-ounce glasses of liquids per day. Water is preferred. However, juices or other cafffeine-free beverages also are solid choices.

Breast-feeding is a technique that is learned. In the early stages it might seem awkward and painful, but with time it can be an enjoyable experience for you and baby. Mothers who are unable to breast-feed for whatever reason, or who simply do not have a desire to breast-feed, can supply adequate nutrition for their infants through balanced infant formulas. Many baby food companies have tried to make their infant formulas as close as possible to mother's milk. However, they haven't been able to duplicate the immunity factors. The positive aspects of bottle feeding are:

■ You have more freedom.

- Dad or other family members can participate in infant feedings (also possible if you pump breast milk or supplement breast-feedings with formula feedings occasionally).

- You have more time in between feedings, because formula takes longer to digest than breast milk.

- You know exactly how much food the baby is getting with each feeding.

- With bottle-fed babies, you might find feeding in public is less stressful.

- There are no dietary or clothing restrictions as there are when breast-feeding.

YOUR DOCTOR'S ADVICE

"I REALLY THINK I need to come into the office," Sally told the nurse. She was feeling some pain, was depressed, and was certain that something must be wrong with her episiotomy. So she made an appointment, went to see her doctor, and found out that everything was fine. Although nothing was medically wrong, she felt much better for having gone to the clinic.

She realized later that the only thing wrong was that she had been cut off from the support systems which had comforted her throughout pregnancy. In fact, what she really needed was just to hear her doctor say everything was okay. That's a perfectly good reason for a postpartum doctor visit. But there are some other, perhaps more serious reasons women definitely need to call their physicians in the early postpartum period:

- Unusual bleeding or hemorrhaging—continuous bleeding which saturates more than one sanitary pad per hour—is a sign that there could be problems. Also, call your doctor if bleeding is bright red any time after the fourth postpartum day, or if your bleeding has faded, and then increases or turns from pinkish to bright red.

Foul odor. If there is a strange odor to your lochia discharge (different from regular menstrual odor), then you need to call the clinic. This could indicate infection. Also, call if you notice large blood clots in your discharge (some small clots are normal).

Temperature. A temperature of more than one hundred degrees for more than twenty-four hours or a temperature of at least 101 degrees for more than three hours could indicate an infection. You should discuss this with your physician or nurse.

Sharp pain. Pain in the chest needs immediate (or even emergency) attention. You also should call if you feel pain and warmth in your calf or thigh, which could indicate a possible blood clot.

Hardening in a localized area of your breast once engorgement has subsided.

Swelling in the perineal area or redness and oozing in your cesarean incision.

Major depression accompanied by violent thoughts of harming yourself or your baby.

Call your doctor if you experience any of the above symptons.

WEIGHT GAIN/WEIGHT LOSS

PHYSICIANS REPORT that the most effective way to speed up recovery after childbirth is to avoid excess weight gain during pregnancy, and to become active as soon as possible after delivery.

A friend of ours was telling us about his wife's pregnancy. He explained that she was in her eighth month and had gained sixty-five pounds.

My husband's response was, "Wow, she's going to have her work cut out for her after delivery."

But this friend said, reassuringly, "Oh, the weight's not fat—it's as hard as a rock! It's all baby."

My husband just smiled and nodded. What could he say? Many of us, myself included, believe during pregnancy that our weight gain is all baby. But unfortunately, we are only going to lose about twelve pounds at delivery.

Weight gain is probably the most frequently discussed topic during pregnancy. It is difficult to say exactly how much weight should be gained during pregnancy. Guidelines have changed over the years. Twenty years ago it was thought that significant restriction of weight gain would prevent toxemia of pregnancy and maternal hypertension. Doctors typically told their patients to gain no more than fifteen pounds. Women who followed that recommendation were having six-pound babies, but they would come out of pregnancy looking much like they did before, except for a loss in muscle tone.

Babies whose mothers gained less than twenty pounds during pregnancy also had a greater chance of being premature and small for gestational age, and of suffering growth retardation in the uterus. In addition, it was revealed that restricting weight gain to fifteen pounds was not preventing toxemia. The only tangible benefit was that the mother was left with less fat to lose.

On the other hand, too much weight gain causes difficulties with assessment and measurement of the fetus, and many other problems for the mother. Among those problems are musculoskeletal pain, varicose veins, an oversized baby that is difficult to deliver vaginally, postpartum obesity, and unhappiness.

In the 1970s, it was determined that a sensible and optimal weight gain for the average woman is between twenty and twenty-seven pounds.[4] This weight range reflects the physiological weight gain of pregnancy, which is the weight gain needed for

---

[4]R. Naeye, "Weight Gain and the Outcome of Pregnancy." *American Journal of Obstetric Gynocology.* (Mosby Year Book: St. Louis, Missouri; 1979); Food and Nutrition Board, Commission on Maternal Nutrition. "Maternal Nutrition and the Course of Human Pregnancy." (National Academy of Sciences, Washington, D.C., 1992)

an optimal pregnancy. That means if you gained twenty-seven pounds during pregnancy, most of that weight is directly related to the pregnancy, and not to excess fat. The following is a breakdown of the approximate distribution of the twenty-seven pounds:

BABY	7 1/2 POUNDS
PLACENTA	1 1/2 POUNDS
AMNIOTIC FLUID	2 POUNDS
UTERINE ENLARGEMENT	2 POUNDS
MATERNAL BREAST TISSUE	2 POUNDS
MATERNAL BLOOD VOLUME	3 POUNDS
FLUIDS IN MATERNAL TISSUE	3 POUNDS
MATERNAL FAT	6 POUNDS

By following the recommendation for a twenty- to twenty-seven-pound weight gain, you should experience a quicker return to your prepregnancy weight. However, everyone is different, and women who begin pregnancy underweight might need to gain more, while those who begin pregnancy overweight might safely gain less. Your doctor is the best judge of the optimal weight gain for you. But no matter how much you gain, with a little work and a sound exercise program, you will lose the fat you want to after delivery.

The average rate of weight increase for women should be about three to four pounds during the first trimester, and about one pound a week during the second trimester and during most of the third trimester. In the ninth month, weight gain might drop off to only a couple of pounds for the month. It is not necessary for a woman to follow this pattern of weight gain precisely. The goal should be to keep weight gain as steady as possible without sudden increases or decreases. You should follow your doctor's recommendations.

■ ■ ■ ■ ■ ■ ■

The average rate of weight increase for women should be about three to four pounds during the first trimester, and about one pound a week during the second trimester and during most of the third trimester.

If you have already delivered or are about to deliver, and your weight gain during pregnancy did not go according to plan, don't be discouraged. You can lose excess babyfat with the Body Contouring Program. We've worked with women who had as many as five children and had not lost their excess pregnancy fat after any of their pregnancies. That means they had an excess of about seventy-five or eighty pounds to lose. (And they did it!) It might simply take longer to achieve your goals if you have more fat to lose.

If you are in the final stages of pregnancy and have gained too much weight, now is not the time to begin restricting nutrients. Monitor your diet carefully and avoid excessive fatty foods, but never restrict calories during pregnancy without being under strict supervision of your doctor. The baby requires a daily supply of nutrients.

■ EXERCISE AFTER DELIVERY

"I NEVER DREAMED I could feel so ugly and so undesirable as I did after that day," Sheryl explained in a Bye-Bye Babyfat class. Her baby was two months old, and Sheryl had taken him to the pediatrician for a check-up. The nurse weighed the baby, then handed him back to Sheryl and said, "You are nursing him too often. He is getting a little chubby, and we don't want him to end up overweight like his mommy now, do we?"

Sheryl said she burst into tears and could hardly even speak when the doctor came in. When she told him what the nurse had said, he tried to reassure her. But the damage was done. "I dwelled on what that nurse said twenty-four hours a day for the next few months," Sheryl said. "I knew I was overweight, but I didn't know what to do about it. I was thin before my pregnancy and I thought I would just naturally get my figure back afterwards. It wasn't until about a year after my son was born that I realized it wasn't going to happen naturally. I tried getting make-overs and new hairstyles, but nothing made me feel any better. I wanted my figure back, and I didn't know how to do it," she explained.

Eventually, Sheryl was successful at losing fat and toning her body. Since she didn't begin our program until one year after delivery, she continued to put on excess fat during the weeks and months after her baby was born. By the time she began exercising, she had an extra forty pounds of fat to lose. Immediately after delivery, she would have only had about twenty-five pounds to lose.

Exercise is one of the most critical components of postpartum recovery. It is the most effective way to facilitate the speediest possible recovery from childbirth. The problem is knowing what kind of exercise to do and how it works to give you the results you want.

> *Exercise is one of the most critical components of postpartum recovery.*

American society is years behind other industrialized countries in providing well-defined exercise programs that meet the needs of postpartum women. Our Body Contouring Program has been shown to reduce body fat, improve energy levels, self-esteem, and appearance, and help reduce stress. This program has been designed specifically for postpartum women, and it gives you step-by-step guidelines that are simple and easy to follow.

Any successful exercise program must be designed to fit the needs of the individual by taking into consideration her desires, condition, and motivation. That's why our program begins by helping you develop effective coping skills and techniques which will help ensure your success in meeting your health, fitness, and appearance goals.

CHAPTER FOUR

Is this the Body You're Stuck With?

s I lay in my hospital bed the night after Michael was born my stomach felt flat. It was a great feeling to have my body back again, and I couldn't wait to jump on the scales and see my weight hovering back down around 120 pounds.

The next morning I walked down the hall of the hospital to weigh myself. I stepped on the scales, and stood there in disbelief. "They have to be broken," I assured myself. But they weren't. How could I possibly still weigh 140 pounds? I thought my weight gain was "all baby." I ate healthy food and exercised regularly throughout my pregnancy. How could I be left twenty pounds heavy?

I stood in front of my hospital mirror, and the image looking back at me didn't look like someone who had just had a baby. It looked like someone who was six months pregnant. What was going on? When I was lying in bed my stomach was flat. But when I stood up, this big bulge just plopped out in front. How could my abdomen have felt so flat immediately after delivery, yet be protruding so far out the next day? The pain from my incision seemed to be intensifying and overtaking my enthusiasm about the birth of my baby.

I was exhausted, I felt unattractive, I was in pain, and I felt an emptiness inside my body where new life had been for the previous forty weeks. My feelings toward my body were confusing and negative, as though it had betrayed me, and my identity was changing. I felt so disillusioned.

*E*ven with a background in weight management, self-esteem enhancement, and stress management, this was a difficult transition for me. I began to review what I knew about body image. One's body image is a picture of his or her body seen through the mind's eye. It is a product of the imagination. We create our body image based on what we see, how we think about what we see, how we feel about it, how we control it, and what other people have said to us over time. That's why having a baby has such an impact on a woman's body image. It changes the way her body looks, the way she thinks and feels about her body, how her bodily functions work, and the way others view her.

Think about it. Having a baby affects your body image in every category.[5]

■ Visually—what you see when you look at yourself

■ Mentally—how you think about what you see

■ Functionally—how your body performs various functions (bowel and bladder function, etc.)

■ Socially—how others see and respond to you

This is important, because there is a strong connection between body image and self-esteem. If your body image is negative, your self-esteem will suffer and this will affect your ability to function and cope as a new mother. High self-esteem is a critical component in one's ability to manage stress. It's easy to develop a negative body image after having a baby. Your body is carrying extra weight; it might appear saggy and flabby; you are in pain; and many of your bodily functions such as bladder and bowel control might be temporarily altered. This also is a time when you might get a great deal of feedback from others regarding your appearance (both verbally and nonverbally).

---

[5] R. Freedman, *Bodylove: Learning to Like Our Looks and Ourselves.* (Harper and Row: New York., 1988)

Jan, a postpartum patient, came to see me six weeks after her daughter was born. She weighed more than two hundred pounds and wanted to begin a program to get back in shape. This was her fifth child, and she had attempted unsuccessfully to lose her excess pregnancy weight after each child was born. She had not gained all of her excess weight at once, but had failed to lose the fifteen pounds of excess fat after each pregnancy. Multiplied by five, she had gained in excess of seventy-five pounds of fat.

Jan was in tears when she first entered my office and related an experience which had occurred the previous week. She was in a department store and a sales clerk enthusiastically asked her when her baby was due. The baby, at home with her father, had been born five weeks earlier. Even though the clerk meant no harm, her comment pierced Jan to the core. Her emotional pain was evident, as she related other experiences which had severely damaged her body image, her self-esteem and her ability to function. By using our Body Contouring Program and practicing the coping techniques recommended in this book, Jan was successful in reaching her goals. She was able to rebuild her self-esteem, restructure her body image, and lose her excess fat.

Many women experience similar painful remarks during the postpartum period. Since we are so vulnerable to the critical glances and to the comments of others during this time, how can we avoid the negative body image and negative self-esteem cycle which affects so many of us? There is a way, and it involves self-understanding, effective coping, and a positive plan for self-improvement.

FEELING GOOD ABOUT YOUR BODY ■

IT IS IMPORTANT TO REMEMBER that while your negative feelings about your body image are real, they are not always based on absolute truth. Feelings don't just appear out of thin air, but they arise from your thought processes. If you look in the mirror and focus on negative thoughts about yourself, your body image and your self-esteem will suffer. But if you can learn rational, realistic, and self-enhancing ways of thinking about yourself, your body image and self-esteem will be improved.

When you look in the mirror, learn to focus on thoughts about the miraculous accomplishment your body has just made. Also, think about how quickly you will be back in shape by following a healthy, balanced program. Think of the possibilities for improvement. Refuse to dwell on negative thoughts about the extra weight you are carrying, or about your protruding stomach. Acknowledge that the excess weight and stretched stomach muscles were necessary for developing new life, and were a critical part of this miraculous accomplishment. Focus on the steps you are already taking to regain body shape and tone, and to become the best you can be now that your baby is here.

■ ■ ■ ■ ■ ■

When you look in the mirror, learn to focus on thoughts about the miraculous accomplishment your body has just made.

Also, it's helpful to look at your body logically, not emotionally, and appreciate the process it has been through in developing a new life. It helps to understand the physiological effects of having a baby, and how you can work to regain your shape.

In the following chapters, you will learn about postpartum bodily adjustments that occur naturally, such as the shrinking of your uterus; and other adjustments (such as the tightening of your stomach muscles) which you must work hard to accomplish. Plus, you will learn the positive steps you can take to optimize your health and appearance. It is important to remember that you are in control of much of what happens in the postpartum period—much more so than in labor and delivery.

Accepting and acting on this control that you have is an important first step in optimizing your physical and mental health. People who perceive the most stress in their lives are the ones who perceive the least control over them, as we've discussed before. The more power and control you take over your life, health, weight, muscle tone, and appearance, the more confidence you will have. That confidence will further enhance your self-esteem and your ability to maximize your health and appearance.

WILL YOU EVER BE THE SAME? ■

ONE THING I KNOW FOR CERTAIN is that you will never be the same after having a baby. Babies change everything. But the good news is you can be healthier and more attractive than you've ever been. Having a baby can enrich every part of your life if you let it. You experience more fulfillment, genuine love, and affection than you ever dreamed possible. You experience the true joy of watching another human being—a part of you—grow and develop. Your energy and activity level can be greater than ever, and you have the opportunity to look and feel your very best.

Health educators say that the prevention of physical and mental health problems is far more desirable than dealing with those problems after they occur. The earlier you gain the knowledge and skills necessary to make health-enhancing decisions, the greater your chances of experiencing optimal health and wellness.

There are many fitness and weight-loss programs available to the general public, but most of them leave out one of the most important components—the mental aspect of fat loss. Knowing the steps you should take and preparing yourself mentally for long-term success requires positive self-esteem and effective coping skills. That is why so many programs allow people to experience short-term weight loss, but the weight is re-gained soon after. These programs fail to teach people how to be successful long-term, and that means teaching them how to understand themselves, how to cope, and how to lose body fat permanently.

Women need additional resources and support in order to make the necessary adjustments during the postpartum period. The apparent lack of support provided for women in the early postpartum period has been called the greatest failure in obstetric care. Do not hesitate to call your obstetrician's office and discuss with the nurse or physician any problems or concerns you have.

It is quite common to experience a variety of physical and emotional symptoms during the early postpartum period. Symptoms vary from woman to woman depending on the type of delivery (easy or difficult, vaginal or cesarean) and other factors. Physically, you might experience a bloody vaginal discharge called lochia which will turn pinkish after approximately one week, as well as abdominal cramps or afterpains as the uterus contracts.

You might have perineal pain (in the area between the vagina and the rectum), especially if you had stitches, incision pain if you had a cesarean, exhaustion, difficulty urinating for a couple of days, and difficulty with bowel movements. In addition, it is common to experience general achiness, bloodshot eyes, and possible bruising on various parts of the body. Perspiration, breast discomfort and engorgement, and sore or cracked nipples are common symptoms as well. Most of these symptoms will disappear in the first week or two, at which time your primary physical complaints will likely be fatigue or exhaustion, excess weight, and other appearance concerns.

Postpartum emotional symptoms might last longer, depending on the coping resources you utilize. Feelings of elation and depression, and swings between the two are common. Many women report intense emotions, both happiness and sadness, during the postpartum period. Deep thinking about issues such as the meaning of life, love, and relationships is common. Fear and concern about mothering, breast-feeding, and regaining a sense of control over your life is typical as well. Women often report feeling overwhelmed, ignored, lonely, isolated, bored, unattractive, irritable, indecisive, angry, resentful, and weepy.

Another of my clients, Teresa, was a case in point. "I can't stand myself," Teresa said, as I spoke with her by phone. "I heard that you help women who are having problems after childbirth, and I need you to help me. I feel fat and ugly, and I don't know what else to do. I've tried getting make-overs, new clothes, and a new haircut, and nothing helps."

We scheduled an appointment, and when Teresa walked through my office door, I saw a very attractive, very groomed young woman who looked like she'd recently had a baby. She told me that ever since her baby was born three months earlier, she had been feeling terrible about the way she looked. After being thin her whole life, she said she could not adjust to her larger postpartum body, and she had been unsuccessful at losing the excess fat. As we continued to talk, Teresa explained that her husband's family told her she was unattractive, and their painful comments had destroyed her self-esteem. I found it hard to believe that they actually told this beautiful woman she was unattractive, so I asked her to explain.

"We were at a family reunion a few weeks ago, and my husband's mother said she was so happy that our son looked like his father," she explained. "What she was really saying is that she was so happy he doesn't look ugly like me." As she told this story, I realized that since Teresa had not yet lost her pregnancy weight and was feeling unhappy with herself, and because she was fatigued and overstressed, she was perceiving things in a negative way.

Looking at the situation from an objective point of view, it was only natural for Teresa's in-laws to think the new baby looked like their side of the family. They were not implying that Teresa was unattractive or that they didn't want the baby to look like her. Instead, they were seeing the baby as a continuation or a new branch of their family tree. I asked Teresa who her parents thought the baby resembled, and she answered, "My parents think he looks like me."

After a few weeks on our Body Contouring Program, Teresa began to regain her shape, and she learned new ways of managing stress. She looked back on this story and laughed. "I can see now how irrational it was for me to take their comments personally, but at the time I was positive that by saying our baby looked like my husband, they were criticizing me because I was fat," she explained.

Many of us have experiences similar to Teresa's during the

postpartum period. It sometimes seems like we are looking at the world through a pair of dark-colored glasses. Our perceptions are altered due to stress and fatigue. The important thing to remember during this stressful time is that things might seem worse than they are, and that you will get yourself back together.

As you realize your tendency to perceive things more negatively, you will be able to recognize irrational thinking when it first begins. This will spare you a great deal of stress. It will not happen overnight, but with time and effort on your part, you will be headed for the most joyous phase of your life.

5
CHAPTER FIVE

Your Pre-Conditioning Activity Program

*I*deally, with your doctor's consent, your Pre-Conditioning Program will begin about one day after delivery. However, if it has been a few weeks, months, or even years since your baby was born and you are now wanting to shape up, you should also complete the Pre-Conditioning Program before you begin the Body Contouring Program. The Pre-Conditioning Program has three components: 1) paced walking; 2) pelvic and abdominal toning exercises; and 3) lower-extremity exercises. The program schedule for walking is located at the end of this chapter.

GETTING STARTED ■

IT'S ONE THING to talk about the benefits of getting up and walking soon after delivery, and another to actually do it. "Ouch, I'm not ready yet!" I groaned as the nurse attempted to help me get up and walk to the bathroom. It had been about ten hours since Michael was born. I was only moderately uncomfortable as long as I lay in one position and did not move.

Intellectually, I knew all the reasons why I really needed to get up. But emotionally, it felt like all my internal organs would fall out on the floor the moment I stood up. The nurse and Mike helped me gradually sit up in bed, and then stand up. It seemed to take forever just to reach the standing position.

I walked a couple of steps and then sat back down on the bed. "How can something that feels so bad actually be so good for me?" I said. I remember asking that question over and over. The fact is, in most cases, walking within the first several hours after delivery is very beneficial. Ideally, you should be out of bed and walking in your room within twelve hours after delivery. However, this depends on the type of delivery you had and the type of medication you were given. For example, many physicians request that patients who received spinal anesthesia remain flat on their backs for eight to twelve hours after delivery to avoid leakage of fluid from the puncture site and to reduce the likelihood of spinal headache.

Early walking helps stimulate circulation, which reduces stiffness and pain. It encourages kidney, bladder, and intestinal activity; facilitates healing of the traumatized uterus; promotes uterine tone; facilitates drainage of lochia and expulsion of clots; helps prevent thrombophlebitis (blood clots in the veins of the legs); and helps to more quickly eliminate anesthetic substances from a woman's system. Even for a healthy individual, a few days of being immobilized is debilitating.

■ ■ ■ ■ ■ ■ ■

Early walking helps stimulate circulation, which reduces stiffness and pain.

It is much more important for a patient who is recovering to become active, so she doesn't begin to suffer even more from the debilitating effects of being bedridden. During your hospital stay, always request assistance before getting up and walking—even to the restroom. Dizziness is commonly experienced during the early postpartum period. It might be caused by dilation of blood vessels, by decreased intraabdominal pressure, pooling of blood in the vessel of the gut, and by excessive blood losses during delivery.

When you get up to walk, it is important to practice good body mechanics (body alignment). Pelvic joint instability and overstretched stomach muscles put the lower back at risk and cause a feeling of looseness in the joints. We suggest:

■ Having someone help you get out of bed by rolling you onto your side, with hips and knees flexed.

■ Pushing yourself up into a sitting position by using your arms and allowing your legs to dangle over the side of the bed.

You should try to stand as straight as possible, with your weight equally distributed on both feet and balanced between the heels and balls of your feet.

Your knees should be flexible (slightly bent), not in a locked position. Your shoulders should be relaxed.

Your abdominal muscles should be slightly contracted and your pelvis in the "neutral" position, not tilted forward or back.

In addition to early walking, postpartum recovery exercises (movements designed to help the mother regain optimal physical condition) should be done as soon after delivery as your doctor permits. Recovery exercises are important for minimizing or even preventing certain complications, and for providing a foundation from which the mother can work to maximize her physical health. The primary function of these exercises is to:

regain proper alignment of the pelvic girdle;

regain function of the abdominal and pelvic floor muscle groups;

regain proper placement of the pelvic organs;

regain energy levels necessary for burning excess body fat;

prepare the mother for future physical exercise necessary to regain optimal body shape and tone.

Poor alignment of the pelvic girdle can lead to postural problems such as neck and shoulder problems and improper breathing. Weaknesses in pelvic floor muscles can lead to poor urinary control, prolonged discomfort, hemorrhoids, prolapse (falling) of pelvic organs, a weakened low back, and can interfere with normal sexual relations. Weak abdominal muscles contribute to poor posture and lower back problems. The following exercises have been shown to be beneficial in restoring optimal function in all of the areas previously mentioned.

KEGAL (PELVIC FLOOR) EXERCISES

KEGAL EXERCISES STIMULATE CIRCULATION to promote healing, relieve pain, alleviate stiffness and edema, and encourage return of bladder control so that you don't leak urine. These exercises help in the shrinkage of hemorrhoids and assist in re-establishing support of the pelvic organs.

Like your abdominal muscles, your pelvic floor muscles will not regain tone naturally. You must exercise them. Kegals are the optimal exercises for these muscles. They are convenient to perform, and might be done in almost any position.

■ A preferred position is to lie on your back, with your head on a pillow and with a pillow beneath your knees.

■ Gently contract your pelvic floor muscles (around the vagina) while also tightening the sphincters (around the anus). The muscles you are trying to contract are those which are involved as you attempt to stop the flow of urine.

If you're not sure how to do this exercise, sit on the toilet and begin to urinate, then attempt to stop midstream. Release a little more urine and stop again. That is the way a Kegal should feel. After delivery, your muscles have lost so much tone that you might not be able to stop your urine flow when you try Kegals. Don't be discouraged. The purpose of the exercise is to help restore that muscle tone. Even if you barely reduce the flow of urine when you attempt to do a Kegal exercise, you are doing what is necessary to begin the process of regaining tone.

As you continue to do Kegals, you will notice your muscles getting stronger. You will be able to cut off more and more of your urine flow. The contractions should be held gently for one to three seconds, and then completely released. Repeat these as often as you feel comfortable. The more you do Kegals, the more you will improve muscle tone and function in your stretched perineal area. It is helpful to do Kegals periodically throughout the day. Once you know how they feel, you can do the exercises lying in bed, standing in the shower, or sitting on the couch.

The reason we recommend doing the exercises first while urinating is that by attempting to cut off your urine flow, you will understand exactly how a Kegal exercise feels, and you will be able to observe the muscles getting stronger. Often, you won't realize how weakened and stretched your perineal muscles have become until you attempt to do Kegals while urinating. (You might find that it's difficult to cut off urine flow.) This helps you realize how much work you need to do.

Many women who don't realize the importance of doing these exercises never regain their perineal tone. In those cases, they have urine-leaking problems for the rest of their lives. One of our clients has had five babies and no one ever told her about Kegal exercises or the need to regain perineal tone. She would leak urine when she tried to do any type of physical exertion, thinking this was a condition she was just stuck with.

When I explained to her that she had never regained her pre-pregnancy muscle tone, she began to do our postpartum exercises (even though it had been twenty-five years since she had her last baby). In time, she regained much of her muscle tone and now walks three miles a day and has no problem with leaking urine. Although it's best to tone up right after delivery—it's never too late to begin.

PELVIC REALIGNMENT EXERCISES (P-R EXERCISES)

THESE EXERCISES HELP STRENGTHEN AND TIGHTEN the muscles that realign the pelvis back into proper position. During pregnancy, our abdominal muscles are stretched out, while the muscles in our lower backs tend to tighten from being overworked and overused. The P-R exercises will help strengthen the abdominal muscles. If you don't begin an exercise program designed specifically to strengthen these muscles, you will begin to experience muscle atrophy and tissue degeneration. To perform these exercises, lie on your side or on your back with pillows supporting your head and knees. Get into a comfortable position, and get ready to reclaim your beautiful, toned body!

Abdominal Squeeze

THIS EXERCISE FOCUSES on tightening and shortening those stretched abdominal muscles. When you first start doing abdominal squeezes, your muscles will be very weak. You will probably notice the muscles shaking as you begin to use them. Don't be alarmed. A muscle that is stretched out, like our abdominals are after pregnancy, is very weak.

Think about the biceps muscle in your upper arm. When your arm is straight, hanging down by your side, your biceps muscle is stretched out. If someone handed you a heavy weight and asked you to curl it up to your chest, you would have a difficult time doing it. However, if your biceps muscle is shortened or contracted a little (as it is when your elbow is bent), you could probably handle the heavy weight.

The point is that muscles are weak when they are stretched out. We want to shorten the abdominals so they can help support your weight, help provide you with an attractive, flat stomach, and prevent or eliminate back problems.

Now, let's begin:

- You are lying on your back, with your knees bent and supported underneath by a pillow.

- Inhale deeply, and then slowly exhale as you tighten your abdominal muscles. This breathing technique is very important for all of these toning exercises, since you might have a tendency to hold your breath during muscle contractions. Always exhale as you contract your muscles.

- Place your hand on top of your abdominals and feel the contraction. Hold the contraction for about three to five seconds (exhaling as you hold), and then release.

Repeat this exercise five times. Remember, since your abdominal muscles have been stretched and weakened during pregnancy, don't be surprised if they quiver or shake as you hold the contraction. Your muscles will shake less as they become stronger. As you become more comfortable doing these exercises, you can lift your head and curl up slightly during the contraction. Make sure your shoulders remain on the bed, or no more than an inch or two high if you lift them.

Abdominal-Pelvic-Hip Squeeze

THIS EXERCISE WORKS YOUR ABDOMINALS, your perineal muscles in the vaginal area, and your buttocks muscles.

If you've had a vaginal delivery, with or without an episiotomy, these muscles have been extremely stretched. Remember, these are the muscles responsible for holding urine, for supporting your female organs, and for providing some degree of sexual pleasure. Strengthening your buttocks muscles helps to strengthen your perineals.

- Begin in the same position as you were during the abdominal squeezes—lying on your back with your knees slightly bent. Contract your abdominals and your pelvic floor muscles at the same time.

■ Now, inhale, and then as you exhale, tighten your abdominals and your pelvic floor muscles (the sensation is as if you were cutting off the flow of urine). Hold the contraction for three to five seconds (as you exhale) and release. Do this five times with the abdominals and the perineals, and then do five more adding the gluteals (buttocks).

■ Use the same breathing techniques, only this time contract the abdominals, the pelvic floor muscles, and the gluteals at the same time. Squeeze your buns together as if you were attempting to hold a quarter in between them, without letting it drop. Hold for three to five seconds and release.

These exercises involve a tightening or contraction of the three major muscle groups which control the pelvis—the abdominals, the pelvic floor muscles, and the gluteals. During pregnancy, as these muscle groups are stretched, women are typically drawn into a posture with a curve in the low spine (lordosis) and a protruding lower abdomen. You might observe that most women who have had babies have a pooch in the lower abdominal area. Most of us would like to have a nice, flat stomach.

After childbirth, it is essential to do these exercises if you want a flat stomach. Flat, tight abdominal muscles take a little work and effort on your part, but if you'll do these exercises regularly, you'll be on your way to having a flat stomach and great posture, too. You will practically eliminate your risks of experiencing chronic, low-back pain as well. (Back pain is quite common for women who don't exercise after childbirth.)

Lower-Extremity Exercises

LOWER-EXTREMITY EXERCISES will help you stimulate circulation to your legs and feet. This will prepare you for your walking program. There are four lower-extremity exercises that have been shown to be helpful after childbirth. You can do these four exercises while lying comfortably on your back.

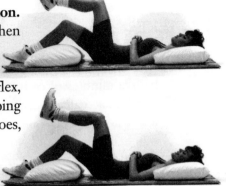

- **Ankle flexion and extension.** Point your toes gently, and then flex your foot. Repeat this exercise ten times (point and flex, one, point and flex, two...). If any muscle cramping occurs while pointing your toes, gently flex your foot and hold until the cramping stops.

- **Ankle circles.** Circle the toes and foot in clockwise and then counterclockwise position. Repeat five circles in each direction and with each foot.

- **Contract your quadriceps** (the large muscles in the front of your thigh). Hold the tension for five to ten seconds and repeat ten times. Do not lift your legs off the bed. These muscles are important for keeping the knees strong when you are standing.

- **Leg bends.** Finally, bend one knee and draw one heel up gradually toward the buttock while inhaling, and then slide the leg out straight while exhaling. This exercise should be repeated five times with each leg. Note: Keep heel on the mat when exercising immediately after the delivery.

Try to do the Kegal and pelvic floor exercises every hour, and the lower extremity exercises about three times per day.

◼ WALKING

DURING THE FIRST FEW DAYS AFTER DELIVERY, your goal should be five minutes of continuous walking, two or three times per day. It is actually easier to do your walking in the hospital than it is when you get home. At the hospital, someone is there to watch the baby, and you have access to the long corridors (which are as good as an indoor track for slow walking). The key to success is making the effort. If you get to walk only once a day at first, that's better than not walking at all.

Once you get home, you have several options regarding your walking. You might walk inside on a treadmill, outside by yourself, or outside carrying your baby. Carrying your baby in a front pack while you walk is healthy for you and for the baby. Some studies have shown that infants enjoy this position and will be more content all day long if they are carried around for extended periods of time each day. It is a great bonding time. Also, you will get an even better workout if you carry the baby while you walk. But if you have help, you might want to use your walking time as a time to be alone.

During the second week after delivery you will gradually increase the time of your walks. You might be able to begin walking to the mailbox and back, down the driveway, around the yard, or whatever you can manage depending on how you feel. Gradually increase your time until you can walk for about twenty to thirty minutes comfortably. (Follow our walking schedule at the end of this chapter.)

If it is not convenient for you to get outside and walk, explore other options. Perhaps you could have a friend take you to the mall or to a shopping center. A very good option is to put on some of your favorite music, and with the baby strapped on, do some moderate dancing or moving to music. This is a great form of low-intensity exercise and can be done in your own den or bedroom. The idea is to get up and move around gently and carefully. The more active you can become, the more rapidly you will recover.

Pre-Conditioning Program
Walking Schedule—Week 1

Day 1	❏	5 minutes easy walk, 2 or 3 times per day
Day 2	❏	5 minutes easy walk, 2 or 3 times per day
Day 3	❏	10 minutes easy walk, 1 time per day
Day 4	❏	10 minutes easy walk, 1 time per day
Day 5	❏	Rest day
Day 6	❏	15 minutes easy walk, 1 time per day
Day 7	❏	20 minutes easy walk, 1 time per day

During the Pre-Conditioning Program, walk slowly at a speed you can comfortably maintain without stopping for the prescribed number of minutes. Do not get out of breath. If you feel pain or any unusual symptom while doing any of the recommended exercises, stop and consult your physician!

Pre-Conditioning Exercises
Do These Every Day—Check Off Each Day When Completed

Day	Kegals	Abdominal Squeezes	Hip Squeezes	Four Lower-Extremity Exer.
1	❏	❏	❏	❏
2	❏	❏	❏	❏
3	❏	❏	❏	❏
4	❏	❏	❏	❏
5	❏	❏	❏	❏
6	❏	❏	❏	❏
7	❏	❏	❏	❏

■ Kegals—20 contractions, hold 3 seconds, 3 to 5 times per day.

■ Abdominal Squeezes—5 contractions, 3 times per day.

■ Hip Squeezes—5 contractions, 3 times per day.

■ All Four Lower-Extremity Exercises, once per day.

Obtain your doctor's approval before beginning this program.

PRE-CONDITIONING PROGRAM
WALKING SCHEDULE—WEEK 2

Day 1	❑	20 minutes easy walk
Day 2	❑	25 minutes easy walk
Day 3	❑	15 minutes easy walk
Day 4	❑	20 minutes easy walk
Day 5	❑	Rest day
Day 6	❑	30 minutes easy walk
Day 7	❑	20 minutes easy walk

PRE-CONDITIONING EXERCISES
DO THESE EVERY DAY—CHECK OFF EACH DAY WHEN COMPLETED

DAY	KEGALS	ABDOMINAL SQUEEZES	HIP SQUEEZES	FOUR LOWER-EXTREMITY EXER.
1	❑	❑	❑	❑
2	❑	❑	❑	❑
3	❑	❑	❑	❑
4	❑	❑	❑	❑
5	❑	❑	❑	❑
6	❑	❑	❑	❑
7	❑	❑	❑	❑

■ Kegals—20 contractions, hold 3 seconds, 3 to 5 times per day.

■ Abdominal Squeezes—5 contractions, 3 times per day.

■ Hip Squeezes—5 contractions, 3 times per day.

■ All Four Lower-Extremity Exercises, once per day.

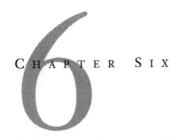

C H A P T E R   S I X

Mommy Sings the "Baby Blues"

*H*aving a baby is one of the greatest experiences in a woman's life. However, it is common and quite normal for mothers to feel sad, afraid, angry, and anxious after childbirth. Many women are surprised at how isolated, fragile, and overwhelmed they feel after delivery. Their feelings do not match their expectations. This disappointment can cause a great amount of stress.

According to the American College of Obstetricians and Gynecologists (ACOG), postpartum blues affect about 70-80 percent of women and can occur after any birth, not just the first. The baby blues involve feelings of unhappiness and other emotions which come and go, and might change hour to hour. Baby blues are alleviated when effective coping strategies are utilized.

Fewer than 10 percent of women develop a more troubling condition after childbirth called postpartum depression, which lasts longer, is more intense, and often requires counseling and treatment. Postpartum depression, a rare condition, is suspected when women are unable to function in their daily routines, and when they have thoughts of harming their babies or themselves. American society offers little guidance and support for women after their babies are born, despite the fact most women desperately need it. This section discusses the baby blues and postpartum depression, factors which contribute to these conditions, and some steps you can take if you feel that you need additional help with postpartum adjustment.

Most women's feelings about the childbirth experience rarely match their expectations. For example, you might feel guilty about feeling down when you expected to feel happy, and you might fear that these feelings mean that you are not a good mother. You might feel angry at the new baby, at your partner, or at other children in the family. You might feel stressed and not even be aware of what is causing your anxiety.

Postpartum blues typically begin about two to three days after birth, and might be triggered by a drop in the hormones estrogen and progesterone after childbirth. Levels of these two hormones are high during pregnancy, and drop drastically after delivery.

Most women's feelings about the childbirth experience rarely match their expectations.

A similar but less dramatic drop in estrogen and progesterone levels happens each month prior to the onset of a woman's menstrual cycle. That monthly drop is believed to be responsible for symptoms associated with premenstrual syndrome (symptoms which are quite similar to postpartum blues). Women are said to experience a type of psychological withdrawal when the levels of these hormones go down. However, adoptive mothers who experience no drastic hormonal fluctuations also report symptoms of the blues and depression. That's why the non-hormonal factors related to the blues and depression, such as exhaustion, lack of sleep, and other stressors, are more likely to be factors in long-term postpartum unhappiness.

With postpartum blues, women might begin to feel sad, weepy, anxious, and moody. It might be difficult to sleep, eat, and make decisions. These feelings come and go after delivery, and might be replaced off and on with feelings of pure joy and happiness.

Kay came to my office explaining that she was at the breaking point. Her husband and her parents believed she was going crazy. She said she was beginning to believe it, too. She wanted me to tell her if I thought she was losing her mind. She had her newborn baby boy with her, and as our conversation progressed, I realized Kay was not crazy at all. She was going through the physical and emotional adjustments of having a new baby, and she was not getting any support or understanding.

At the time, Kay was a thirty-year-old, first-time mother, and her family could not understand why she would become irritated and emotional at what seemed to them like nothing. Her husband felt burdened by her constant need to hear him say how much he loved her, and that he would never leave her. When he would not respond and meet this need she had for security, she would threaten to divorce him and raise the baby on her own.

She explained to me that she didn't even know why she would say these things, because she didn't really want a divorce, but that she would just become overwhelmed with anger. Many new mothers have reported similar feelings. What Kim and other new mothers need from their husbands after the birth of a baby is a sense of security and understanding. Hormonal adjustments and stress make it very difficult to control our moods. If family members understand this, they are better equipped to make allowances for us and support us during this time of hormonal "hell." Women need and deserve a grace period in the weeks following childbirth. We need a time when we are allowed to be ultra-sensitive and emotional, and we need support and encouragement as we regain balance.

The worst thing that can happen to a woman during this time is for her husband or family to respond to her emotional turmoil with condemnation and judgment.

The worst thing that can happen to a woman during this time is for her husband or family to respond to her emotional turmoil with condemnation and judgment. Family members need to make allowances for women until their physical and emotional recovery is complete. This is a great opportunity for a husband to demonstrate his love for his wife by providing stability, and by becoming her anchor in the midst of this storm. He will be more than rewarded for this type of support.

Women can help themselves minimize the effects of postpartum blues by being prepared in advance. Many commonly held beliefs have been shown to contribute to feeling blue. These beliefs might be held by expectant and new mothers.

Some typical statements made by these women might include:

- "If anyone knew how angry and emotional I really feel, he or she would think I am a bad person."

- "If my baby has any problems or gets sick, I will be to blame."

- "There must be something terribly wrong with me if I don't have positive feelings about my baby all of the time."

- "All aspects of motherhood should come easily for me."

- "If I am not constantly joyful about having a baby, there is something wrong with me."

- "My baby always comes first. His desires should take priority over my own needs for eating, exercise, stimulation, and rest."

- "If I can't keep my baby in good spirits most of the time, or if he keeps fussing, I am not being a good mother."

If we understand that these beliefs are destructive, we can attempt to change our thinking. A woman's thoughts and belief systems have a powerful effect in determining her emotional reactions to stressful life situations. Women who have the most difficult time during the postpartum period are those who think in negative patterns about themselves, their circumstances, and others (many of us do this unless we have been taught otherwise). They have a tendency to view ambiguous situations in a pessimistic fashion and are more likely to give up than to try to improve their moods and their lives. If they are not supported and instructed about how to think more functionally, postpartum depression or long-term postpartum stress might result.

Although it is very rare, some postpartum women go into a state of true depression, and these women need psychological help. Following is a description compiled by the American College of Obstetricians and Gynecologists listing conditions under which a woman who suspects she has postpartum depression should seek professional guidance.

Baby blues (extreme) that don't go away after two or three weeks, or strong feelings of depression and anger that begin to surface one to two months after childbirth.

Feelings of sadness, doubt, guilt, helplessness, or hopelessness that seem to increase with each week and begin to disrupt a woman's normal functioning. The woman might not be able to care for herself or her baby. She might have trouble handling her usual responsibilities at home or on the job.

Not being able to sleep even when tired, or sleeping most of the time, even when the baby is awake.

Marked changes in appetite.

Loss of interest in things that used to bring pleasure.

Extreme concern and worry about the baby, or lack of interest in or feelings for the baby; the woman might feel unable to love her infant or her family.

Anxiety or panic attacks—the woman might be frightened of being left alone in the house with the baby.

Fear of harming the baby—these feelings are almost never acted on by women with postpartum depression, but they can be very frightening and might lead to guilty feelings, which only make the depression worse.

Thoughts of self-harm, including suicide.

Since true postpartum depression occurs so infrequently, we will deal primarily with the commonly experienced postpartum blues and long-term postpartum stress. There are many factors believed to contribute to the blues and to feelings of unhappiness. Understanding these factors is important in helping women recognize their own feelings.

First of all, the end of pregnancy can cause feelings of sadness. Many women enjoy being pregnant and all the attention and joy they experience. Especially if this is your first baby, pregnancy is a simple time in which your responsibilities are few and the amount of positive attention you receive is great. Once you deliver, you might feel a sense of loss and emptiness, a sense of being overwhelmed, and you might miss the miraculous sensation of carrying your baby inside your body.

Often, women experience a feeling of anticlimax, because the big event for which they have trained for nine months is now over. There might be feelings of jealousy because all of the attention which has been focused upon you during pregnancy is shifted to the new baby. You might experience feelings of disappointment in your newborn because he/she is so unresponsive. It is common to feel anxious about the responsibilities that face you when you go home from the hospital.

Exhaustion due to delivery, caring for a newborn, and lack of sleep can lead to blues or depression. You might also be experiencing pain and concern about getting your body back to normal. For many women who do not adopt a program for improvement, unhappiness due to your appearance and body function might be a problem for months or even years after childbirth.

▉ REASONS FOR POSTPARTUM UNHAPPINESS
A Summary

RESEARCH IS NOT CLEAR as to why so many of us become unhappy after childbirth. One important factor is physiology. The physical changes which take place after childbirth, such as a drop in the level of maternal hormones, have a tendency to affect a woman's mood and behavior for days or weeks. During the first few days after delivery, estrogen and progesterone levels drop drastically, while the nursing hormones—prolactin and oxytocin—rise sharply. Physical discomforts such as perineal pain, breast engorgement, afterpains, and constipation might also be factors.

It is difficult to be in a good mood when you are in pain. Environmental aspects, such as feelings of isolation, stress, and lack of support from family and friends might also contribute to feeling blue. Finally, according to the American College of Obstetricians and Gynecologists, psychological factors such as low self-esteem and lack of effective coping skills play major roles in the degree to which a woman experiences the blues.

Postpartum blues likely result from a combination of these factors. For each woman, the combination of factors is unique, because no two women have the same physiological make-up, environmental circumstances, or psychological considerations. That probably explains why some women develop postpartum blues to a greater degree than others. It might also explain why some women, who successfully cope with everyday life, find the stress of a new baby is difficult to handle.

The postpartum period is a time of great change in the body. Much smaller decreases in the hormones estrogen and progesterone are experienced by women each month prior to their menstrual periods; they cause symptoms that have contributed to premenstrual syndrome. Because some women are more sensitive to these changes than others, they might be more likely to experience postpartum blues. Thyroid levels might also drop sharply after birth. A new mother might develop a thyroid deficiency, which has been shown to produce symptoms which mimic depression, such as mood swings, severe agitation, fatigue, insomnia, and tension.

Many women suffer from exhaustion after labor and delivery, and it might take weeks to regain normal strength and

> It is difficult to be in a good mood when you are in pain. Environmental aspects, such as feelings of isolation, stress, and lack of support from family and friends might also contribute to feeling blue.

stamina. This might be especially true for women who have cesarean births. New mothers seldom get much-needed rest due to many visitors and interruptions from baby's feedings. Fatigue and lack of sleep might go on for months, and both have been associated with feelings of depression.

Many women have low self-esteem. This affects their ability to handle stress or cope. Having a baby is probably one of the most stressful experiences in one's life, and it is a critical time to develop new coping skills and new ways of managing stress. Also, feelings of loss are very common after childbirth and can contribute to depression. The loss might be experienced as loss of freedom and feelings of being tied down or trapped, loss of an old identity, loss of feeling in control, loss of a slim figure, and loss of feelings of sexual attractiveness.

Finally, lack of emotional support from a partner, relatives, and friends is a major factor in postpartum depression. If a woman is single, divorced, or unmarried, and if she is living away from other family, support might be lacking. This leads to feelings of isolation and overwhelming exhaustion. Remember, if you feel like you need professional help in sorting through confusing and painful feelings, your doctor can refer you to someone trained to help you. For women with postpartum depression, realistic goals and emotional support are important for recovery.

Small changes make a big difference—things such as understanding and being prepared for what types of feelings you can expect after childbirth, taking time for yourself, learning how to manage postpartum stress, getting out of the house, participating in regular exercise, proper diet, and taking steps to look your best all might play a role in minimizing postpartum unhappiness. Remember, when you look your best, you are more likely to feel in control. Feelings of being in control of one's life have been shown to reduce postpartum blues and long-term stress.

CHAPTER SEVEN

Postpartum Stress: A New Perspective

I sat on the sofa sobbing, unable to make a decision and completely confused as to why I was feeling so out of control. Michael was about eight weeks old and we were supposed to go canoeing with our friend, Don. We were planning to take the baby and let him stay on the riverbank for a few hours with Don's parents. It was almost time to leave and, suddenly, I decided that we could not go. I had never left Michael, and I was afraid he would be traumatized by my absence. If the trip took longer than the scheduled two hours, my breasts would become engorged and I would be in pain until I could feed Michael.

But it would be so much fun to get away for a while, and to be carefree the way I was before Michael was born. I definitely needed a break, even if it was only a couple of hours. We should go. But we can't. I must be responsible now. Anything could happen if I'm not there to protect Michael. "Sweetheart, are you ready?" Mike asked, as he walked into the room. Then he realized something was wrong (again!). "What is the matter?" he asked hesitantly. I had no answer. Everything was the matter, and everything was wonderful. I adored this precious baby and I loved being a mom. But there was a part of life and a part of my personality that seemed to have died, and I desperately missed it. Who had I become? Why couldn't I make one single decision and stick with it?

I thought that the "postpartum blues" were supposed to be gone by six weeks after delivery. That's what the pregnancy books said. What I was experiencing didn't feel like depression, but I was definitely not back to normal. Am I going crazy? I asked myself over and over. Am I losing it? My condition, although I didn't realize it at the time, was what I now call postpartum stress, and I believe it can last as long as it takes to complete the various adjustments of having a new baby. For some women who are unable to regain their pre-pregnancy shape, postpartum stress can last for years.

We didn't go on the canoe trip. We stayed home and talked instead. Together, Mike and I decided that we really needed to get away for several days. We decided to take a trip to the beach, together, as a family. That trip turned out to be one of the most valuable postpartum experiences for both of us. Now, that particular beach vacation was nothing like the ones we had taken in the past. There were no romantic, late-night walks along the shore. We had to go in swimming one at a time, and beside our towels in the sand, where frosted drinks and steamy novels used to be, sat baby Michael in a stroller with a beach umbrella and a bottle of No. 25 sunscreen.

Surely, I was not the only woman who experienced continued stress and turmoil after the typically described "six-week" adjustment period. One of my pregnancy books had even suggested that the emotional turmoil would be over in forty-eight hours (it must have been written by a man!). I realized that if I had been prepared, if there would have been something for me to read about postpartum stress, I could have been spared the anxiety of feeling so alone and so abnormal. Many of my postpartum clients have explained to me that one of the most important things they've learned about postpartum adjustment is that they are not alone—that other women are experiencing similar feelings.

STRESS IN THE POSTPARTUM PERIOD

THE POSTPARTUM PERIOD has been described as the greatest failure in obstetric care! That's because not much has been done to help women adapt after a baby is born. The health-care system in the United States has provided less in the way of postpartum care for mothers than any other country. We provide a wealth of information and services for women pertaining to pregnancy and delivery. Most of us attend prenatal classes to become familiar with pregnancy, labor, and birth, and to practice exercises and breathing techniques designed to facilitate labor and delivery. Although these classes are effective in reducing anxiety during pregnancy, as well as in labor and delivery, they do nothing to eliminate the frustrations and the stressors that occur in the postpartum period.

Mothers are being discharged from the hospital after childbirth earlier than ever before. Studies show that new mothers have more questions and concerns during the first few weeks after they go home from the hospital than they have at any other time. Yet it is during this critical period that they are virtually cut off from the medical care system. The new mom's first postpartum checkup is not usually scheduled until the sixth week after delivery. The little postpartum information that is given to a mother comes during her short hospital stay, immediately after the birth of her baby.

The first twenty-four to seventy-two hours after delivery are a poor time for learning. During this time, a mother's priorities are rest, recovery, and physical comfort.

The first twenty-four to seventy-two hours after delivery are a poor time for learning. During this time, a mother's priorities are rest, recovery, and physical comfort. In the United States, most new mothers are discharged within seventy-two hours after delivery. After this seventy-two-hour period, women develop what researchers call a psychological readiness for learning new lifestyle skills and coping strategies. However, it is impossible for us to learn if no information, education, and support is provided during this time. Postpartum stress is real and can be managed effectively if we learn to recognize it and we learn how to cope.

Indeed, the postpartum period is a time of stress overload—labeled by the research as a "crisis period." It is a crisis situation for mothers who must now reorganize their entire lives to include the new baby. They must work through new feelings, manage new stressors, and get themselves back in shape physically (or in shape for the first time). If they fail to make these adjustments effectively, mothers will have to live with unresolved feelings and an out-of-shape body. In other words, they will not have completed postpartum adjustment.

Many women report feeling unprepared to make all these necessary changes. Most mothers report problems such as concerns about appearance, feelings of loss of control, loss of sleep, chronic fatigue, and giving up outside employment or other outside interests. These factors are viewed as barriers to optimal postpartum adjustment. They also say they need a program designed specifically to help them know how to adjust.

Many of my clients report feeling like they are going crazy. That's probably the most common complaint. I can relate to these feelings because I experienced them, too. However, I knew deep down that I was not going crazy. I knew that I was in over my head in the sea of postpartum adjustment, and nobody had taught me how to swim through it. In this sink-or-swim predicament, I learned to swim because of my background in stress management and health. But it would have been much easier, and I would have swallowed a lot less water, if I had been offered some instruction.

When I really began to evaluate the postpartum experience, I realized that it was only normal to feel a little crazy. Not only do we as women have all the hormonal adjustments that take place after delivery, but we also have the hormonal changes associated with breast-feeding and the many, many life stressors associated with having a new baby. I have not met one woman who felt anywhere near completely adjusted in the typically described six-week adjustment period after childbirth. I have, however, come in contact with many women who still have not completed postpartum adjustment when their baby is several years old. Why? Postpartum adjustment is not complete until you've learned to effectively cope with the new stressors in your life, and until your body is back in shape. You will have excess stress based on how you feel about yourself and your body image. This stress will cause problems in other areas of your life.

PROBLEMS WITH POSTPARTUM STRESS

STRESS IS DEFINED as our response to the demands of daily living. You experience stress with every change and adaptation in your life. The change might be positive (having a baby), or negative (losing a job). In either case, you must adapt, change, or adjust, and that causes stress. It is important to realize that your response to external events is what causes stress—not the events themselves.

The events in our lives are stressors. They have the potential to cause stress. How you respond or cope with these events in your life determines how much stress you experience. Everybody reacts differently. That explains why some people who live under extreme stressors might be calm and peaceful, and others who have very little stress appear constantly frazzled. It is possible for us to have some control over the amount of stress we experience—simply by managing the way we interpret or think about stressors (events in our lives which are likely to cause stress). In order to do this effectively, we must learn some strategies.

Many of us have never had the opportunity to learn effective coping strategies, and we're stuck with the ones we picked up from our parents or others from our past. The more effective coping strategies that we can learn to use during the postpartum period, the more stress we can tolerate and the more we can enjoy this precious time. We don't want to avoid stress. It's the "spice" of life. But we must cope with stress one way or another, whether it be through destructive means such as avoidance, withdrawal, depression, drug dependence, or overeating—or through constructive means such as exercise, relaxation, positive self-esteem, positive thinking, quiet time, and others.

■ ■ ■ ■ ■ ■ ■

If you didn't have any stressors in your life you would become very bored. Boredom itself causes a great amount of stress.

Is stress bad for you? Not necessarily. If you didn't have any stressors in your life you would become very bored. Boredom itself causes a great amount of stress. Why? When we are bored we have a tendency to think negative thoughts. Our bodies respond to our thoughts as if they are real events. In other words, our thoughts can cause our bodies to experience physical stress responses. A certain amount of stress adds excitement and motivation. An optimal amount of stress that is positively managed actually increases your energy level. However, chronic, unmanaged stress can lead to fatigue, illness, weight gain, depression, exhaustion, and has even been linked to heart disease, cancer, and other illnesses.

Having a baby—whether it's your first, second, or beyond—is certain to cause stress in your life. Therefore, we will discuss the health problems associated with chronic stress. We also will teach you how you can prepare to prevent those problems through effective stress management.

STRESS AND HEALTH

AT EIGHT WEEKS POSTPARTUM, we headed off to the beach with our newborn. We desperately needed to get away. It would be heaven—a stress-free, relaxation vacation.

It was my turn to drive a stretch on our fourteen hour journey, and I was really beginning to unwind. Baby Michael was asleep in the car seat and we were about seven hours down the road. My favorite tape was playing, Mike was in the back seat with the baby, and all was well. I was beginning to feel moments of peace—and I was certain I was becoming my old self again, strong, confident, carefree.

"Bang!" A loud noise clanged from the back seat, and Michael began screaming like I had never heard him scream before. "What happened?" I yelled at Mike as I turned to see for myself. Baby Michael was covered, head to toe, with Diet Coke. "It's okay," Mike assured me. "I accidentally hit the knob on the front seat and it popped the seat up, hit my hand, and my Coke flew up in the air and spilled on the baby."

I don't know if it was the noise or the cold, "fizzy" liquid, but baby Michael was traumatized. I pulled over and the postpartum monster inside of me reared her ugly head. I became very angry at Mike. "This is all I needed! How could you do something so careless?" I snapped. "What are we doing on this trip anyway? I want to turn around and go back. I just can't take this! Am I ever going to be able to trust you to take care of things with the baby for even five minutes?" It was so upsetting to feel that there was no one—not even my own husband—who was able to take the burden of responsibility of protecting and caring for Michael off of my shoulders. Why couldn't Mike watch the baby for a few minutes without something going wrong? Was I the only one who could be trusted with Michael?

Mike had learned by now to be patient with me at times like this. What choice did he have? He knew that he couldn't win an argument with this side of me. We sat on the side of the road for half an hour, and he convinced me to continue on our trip. It would be good for us, he explained. After I calmed down and realized the baby really was okay, guilt begin to set in. Why did I get so angry? Why was everything such a big deal?

> ■ ■ ■ ■ ■ ■ ■
> *G*oing through pregnancy, labor and delivery, and early postpartum recovery depletes all of your stress reserve. You are truly exhausted, in every sense of the word.

Through this experience, I realized something firsthand that I had been teaching my university students for years. Stress is cumulative. Everyone has a certain amount of "reserve" or tolerance for life's stressors. As you dip into that reserve, you might become less and less able to cope. When your reserve is depleted, it takes time to build it back up. Going through pregnancy, labor and delivery, and early postpartum recovery depletes all of your stress reserve. You are truly exhausted, in every sense of the word. It is probably the most depleted state you will ever experience. That's why it takes such a long time after delivery to really adjust.

This works much the same way as a car battery. When a battery is fully charged, it can take a lot of drain. We can start our car, turn on the light, etc. But once a battery is drained below a certain point, it can't withstand anything—it won't even allow us to play the radio. When it gets to that point, it takes time to recharge. A depleted battery won't recharge instantly. When our stress reserves are depleted, it takes time for us to recharge.

It took me the entire week on the beach to feel that I could begin to cope more effectively again. If the Coke incident had happened on the way home, I would have probably handled it a little better.

Most stress is caused by how you think about things. For example, when you watch a violent television program, you experience many stress responses. Your mind causes your body to respond even though it is not a real experience. When you undergo a stress response, your body is actually altered physiologically for greater speed and strength. This is called the "stress response," or the "fight or flight" response. Historically, fight or flight might have been necessary for survival. People needed to hunt for food and, in many cases, fight or flee in order to survive. In modern times, however, most of us get our food off the supermarket shelves. It is usually considered dysfunctional to run from our problems (flight) or to attack someone who irritates us (fight).

We live in a grin-and-bear-it society. Yet our body prepares us to fight or run. It does this by increasing muscle tension, heart rate, blood pressure, perspiration, stroke volume (amount of blood pumped per beat of your heart), stomach acid, blood glucose (sugar), and many other changes. When you constantly build up these stress products, the result is exhaustion, depression, illness, and disease. When we realize that we are becoming exhausted from chronic stress, as is often the case during the postpartum period, we need to take action and make some changes. Otherwise, we are placing ourselves at risk of suffering more serious health problems.

Many of the illnesses from which people suffer are believed to have stress origins. Prolonged stress, such as the kind we typically experience during the postpartum period, needs to be effectively managed so that it doesn't harm our health. Unmanaged stress over long periods of time decreases the ability of our immune systems to function properly. Since the postpartum period is one of the most stressful times in a woman's life, it is a critical time to practice stress management. Doing so might protect your health long-term. People who do not learn to manage stress often suffer from more colds, flu's and infections.

Even diseases such as cancer have been linked to stress. That is because stress decreases the number of T-lymphocytes, or killer cells which destroy abnormal cells prior to their multiplication. In other words, we all have a certain number of diseased cells in our bodies, but a properly functioning immune system is able to attack these cells before they cause problems.

Chronic stress causes our bodies to have fewer "good" cells to fight off the "bad" cells. Stressed people who lack effective coping skills might place themselves at higher risk for developing cancer than those who practice effective coping. Don't be alarmed. Short-term bouts of stress are not going to cause cancer. But chronic stress over long periods of time might increase your risk for developing lifestyle-related diseases.

Another illness believed to be associated with stress is hypertension. Blood pressure and serum cholesterol can increase with chronic stress, which increases the likelihood of stroke and heart disease. Heart attacks are also believed to be associated with stress. Ulcers are associated with stress as well. Stress might cause an increase in norepenephrine, thus shutting down mucous production needed to coat the lining of the stomach. Therefore, hydrochloric acid breaks down the stomach tissue. Stomach upset and diarrhea are also associated with stress, as are migraine headaches, tension headaches, and backaches.

In order to understand how postpartum stress can work against your long-term health, two factors—duration and degree—must be considered. Duration refers to how long your physiology varies from its baseline or normal measures due to stress, and degree refers to how great the variance is from normal measures. Of these two, controlling the duration of stress has been described as the most important for preventing illness. Most of us can tolerate a great deal of stress in our lives, and we can even tolerate major stressors that cause a strong response. What is most important for our health is learning techniques of coping which

In order to understand how postpartum stress can work against your long-term health, two factors—duration and degree—must be considered.

allow our bodies to return to normal functioning between bouts of stress.

The postpartum period is going to be stressful for all women, and there is no way to change that. But we can prevent long-term or chronic stress by learning how to complete postpartum adjustment, and how to get back to normal or optimal functioning. We need frequent "rest" breaks from stress. Health problems occur when we let little daily hassles build up over long periods of time. This makes a great deal of sense when you consider the following analogy.

What if you were to run ten yards as fast as you could without stopping? Immediately when you hit the ten-yard marker, you ran another ten yards as fast as you could, and another, and another, and another? How many could you do without harming your health, or reaching exhaustion? You probably could only do a few with no rest. However, if you rested in between sprints and allowed your physiology to return to normal, you could do many ten-yard sprints.

That is why the postpartum period is so stressful. It is a time when there is so much demand, and the demand is almost constant. If we are not careful, we can find ourselves taking no breaks and suffering negative health consequences. Stress management skills teach us how to take a rest, return our physiology to normal functioning, and become rejuvenated so that we can continue to meet the demands of motherhood and protect our health, too!

THE FATIGUE FACTOR

RESISTANCE TO STRESS is adversely affected by fatigue. When you are tired, you are less able to deal with stress. That's one reason we're vulnerable to long-term stress during the postpartum period—because we are so fatigued. Think about how children respond to stress. Have you ever observed how flexible and happy a well-rested child is? He responds eagerly and shares when another child wants to play with his toys. However, observe the same child in the same circumstance just before nap time—when he is tired—and he would likely throw a temper tantrum. Or have you ever seen a child have a temper tantrum at the grocery store or in a restaurant, and the mother looks up apologetically and says, "He is just tired"? We are not much different from children. Yet when was the last time you yelled and snapped at your husband and he patiently responded, "Honey, you're just tired"?

People don't make allowances for an adult's tired behavior. Yet, much like children, we need to be rested in order to function appropriately. It becomes instantly apparent how vulnerable we become to arguments and friction with our spouses during the postpartum period. Both husband and wife are typically fatigued and sleep-deprived, and at the same time, don't know how to manage all the extra stress!

Typically, new mothers (and fathers) are not aware of how important adequate sleep and rest are after childbirth. In most cases, the mother's labor has gone on for a number of hours and she is physically exhausted from this experience. Remember, labor and delivery is a major physical event, probably more taxing than a marathon or a triathlon, and a mother needs physical and mental recovery.

In many cases, a woman does not sleep well during the final weeks of pregnancy, so she enters the delivery experience in a state of fatigue. And if that's not enough, mothers tend to get fewer hours of sleep during the night after baby is born. Also, they get a different kind of sleep because the normal cycles of light sleep, dreaming (REM) sleep, and deep sleep are constantly interrupted by the baby. It is psychologically upsetting to be awakened frequently—even under normal circumstances. It becomes much more upsetting when we are attempting to recover from childbirth, and our bodies are craving rest and sleep.

The new mother has several options to prevent or reduce severe fatigue problems. One is to go to bed much earlier and to set aside time for naps. She must begin to treat herself like an athlete in training. Athletes plan their daily schedules around maximizing their physical potential. If that means going to bed at 8:00 P.M., then that is what they do. It will probably be helpful to tailor your sleeping patterns around the baby's—to nap when he naps and go to bed when he does.

The new mother has several options to prevent or reduce severe fatigue problems. One is to go to bed much earlier and to set aside time for naps. She must begin to treat herself like an athlete in training.

If you have other children, you might have to call on outside help from family or friends. You might wish to alternate nights with your husband so that he does the night feedings every other night. You sleep in the other room, or wear earplugs, so you are not awakened when he gets up to feed. If you are breast-feeding, you can pump your breasts in advance. The next night, let your husband sleep in the other room or wear earplugs and you do the night feedings. That way, each of you can get some uninterrupted, deep sleep.

Another secret for preventing fatigue is to exercise. Appropriate, low-intensity aerobic exercise will help relieve stress and tension, improve your mood, and promote rapid healing for your body. Exercise allows your body to vent stress buildup through activity. Since stress actually prepares your body for action, exercising is a natural outlet for stress. Mentally, exercise has the effect of clearing your mind and of stimulating positive thoughts. The side effect of this type of exercise is improved sleep.

Here is a summary of strategies to help the new mom prevent severe fatigue which will allow her to better cope with stress:

■ Take naps during the day.

■ Go to be early at night to prepare for night feedings. Alternate with husband if possible.

■ Reduce or eliminate visits from friends and relatives until you are rested, unless they are coming to help.

■ Seek out help with the household chores, meals, etc. Focus on yourself and the baby.

■ Exercise.

■ Be alert to early signs of fatigue, and take action. These include irritability, mood swings, feelings of unhappiness, feeling overwhelmed, negativity, emotional outbursts, etc. When you notice these symptoms, do whatever you must to get more rest. Rely on family and friends.

■ Utilize the strategies for managing stress outlined in chapter 8.

CHAPTER EIGHT

Effective Strategies for Managing Stress

C oping is defined as the process of managing demands (external, such as lack of sleep, or internal, such as negative thinking) that are perceived as stressful, taxing, or exceeding the resources of the individual. Coping requires effort, skills, and resources. Adaptation is similar to coping. It means changing or accepting your circumstances to reduce stress. Effective coping and/or adaptation is essential during the postpartum period, if you want to experience optimal health and well-being. Healthy adjustment during postpartum involves achieving a balance between acceptance of things as they are, the active effort to change the things that you can, and the ability to effectively cope with stress.

Positive coping strategies during postpartum will allow you to: (1) feel good about yourself; (2) feel good about other people; and (3) meet life's previously existing and new demands.

HIGH SELF-ESTEEM

HIGH SELF-ESTEEM is the major determining factor in your ability to cope or manage life stressors during the postpartum period, and at other times as well. Your self-esteem forms the basic framework from which you must work toward developing skills for managing life stressors. It is the single most significant determinant of an individual's behavior.

During the postpartum period, women report an overwhelming deficit in the area of self-esteem. (American women in general suffer from low self-esteem, and the problem is magnified after childbirth.) This low self-esteem is said to be related to negative perceptions or thoughts about body image.

This is very important, because having a baby drastically alters a woman's body image. Until the mother can get back into shape to the point where she feels good about her body, her self-esteem and her ability to manage stress will be greatly impaired.

In order to effectively manage stress, you must learn to love and respect yourself, mentally and physically. This respect enables you to be successful in other areas of your life. High self-esteem is your foundation for everything else you do. Remember, self-esteem, or how you think and feel about yourself, is the major determinant of behavior. It is critical for women to regain a positive body image and positive self-esteem at some point after childbirth. Once this is done, postpartum adjustment is complete.

Defined simply, self-esteem is the judgment a person makes—or feelings she has— about herself. It is the measure of how much a woman likes and approves of herself. A woman's self-esteem is a part of every other feeling which she experiences. In fact, there is no factor more decisive in our psychological well-being and motivation than self-esteem. It involves a combination of self-confidence and self-respect.

Self-esteem is dynamic and ever changing. If you do a great job at something and people compliment you, your self-esteem is probably temporarily enhanced. If you look good, feel energetic, and are looking forward to something special, your self-esteem is again enhanced. But the reverse also is true. If you feel fatigued or you think you are overweight (typical postpartum feelings) your self-esteem suffers. Or, if someone is critical of you in any way, your self-esteem goes down.

A positive, consistent sense of self-esteem comes from learning to respect and appreciate yourself, and to acknowledge your uniqueness as a human being. It comes from actively directing and controlling your thoughts about yourself. It is the habit of thinking more positively about yourself, and a side effect is that you will think more positively about everything and everyone else as well. People with low self-esteem usually think more negatively toward others. The more positively you view yourself, the more positively you view others.

Take an opportunity to acknowledge positive things about yourself. What are the qualities or attributes that make you special and different? Are you honest, funny, compassionate, cheerful, loving, caring, etc.? Think of all your positive qualities and put them on the following list. Include on your list internal qualities, such as the ones mentioned above, and external qualities, or aspects of appearance ("I have a nice smile."), and roles you play, such as being a wife or mother. Every time you find yourself feeling down, look at this list and review the positive things about yourself. Try to become your own best friend.

> *Take an opportunity to acknowledge positive things about yourself.*

POSITIVE THINGS ABOUT ME
PERSONAL LIST

....

....

....

....

....

....

....

....

....

....

....

Another way to permanently enhance your self-esteem is to prioritize all of the different attributes that make up who you are (self-concept). Self-concept is your set of beliefs and images about yourself. Your self-concept contains a wide variety of images and beliefs regarding you. Some are simply statements of fact: "I am a woman." Others refer to less tangible aspects, such as " I am attractive." Most of your ideas and impressions of yourself have come about in two ways—how others have treated you, and what they have told you about yourself.

Although your ideas about who you are make up your self-concept, your ideas about who you should be make up your ideal self. We constantly compare our perceived "as-is" self to our "ideal" self, and the wider the gap between the two, the lower our level of self-esteem. Often we form our ideas of ideal self from pictures of models on magazine covers, or from other media figures. In many cases, the images we idealize are the results of extensive plastic surgeries. It is helpful to be aware of this so that we can be more realistic in our expectations of what we can achieve without surgery, and changes that might require surgical procedures to achieve.

This does not mean that we are advocating cosmetic surgery, but we are acknowledging that some people perceive deficiencies (example: "My nose is crooked.") that cannot be changed naturally. The more closely your perceived self approaches what you consider ideal, the higher your self-esteem. In the space provided, complete the self-concept diagrams.

First, complete the "Me as I Wish to Be" list by writing down all the attributes and descriptions that define exactly what you would consider "ideal." Then complete the "Me I See" list by writing down the attributes and descriptions that define how you feel now. Compare the two and notice areas that you can realistically change. These will be the areas you will focus on in a goal-setting section later in this book. Also, notice things that might be unrealistic or impractical for you to achieve. These are the areas in which you might need to modify your expectations.

Remember, you want to bring your as-is self as close to your ideal self as possible. The more closely these two self-concepts become, the higher your self-esteem.

Remember, set goals for the things you can actually change so as to bring your "as-is" self closer to your "ideal" self. An example would be, "I weigh 150 pounds and I consider 120 pounds ideal for me." But there might be some things that you cannot change, such as, "I'm five feet tall and I consider five-foot-five ideal." For areas that you cannot change, you might want to adapt, or adjust your expectations.

ME I WISH TO BE
PERSONAL LIST

....

....

....

....

....

....

....

....

....

....

....

ME I SEE
PERSONAL LIST

....

....

....

....

....

....

....

....

....

....

■ GETTING TO KNOW YOURSELF

FEW OF US have ever taken the time to really get to know ourselves, and to understand the things we like and dislike about ourselves. This would be helpful, however, because often the things we don't like about ourselves can be changed. Also, if you have problems with low self-esteem, it might be because you are focusing on the negative things and overlooking the positive. In other words, you might be thinking of yourself emotionally and not realistically.

Let's take a closer look at how this works. There are two types of self-esteem—global and specific. Global is the measure of how much you like and approve of your perceived self as a whole. Specific is the measure of how much you like and approve of a certain part of yourself. For example, if you perceive that you have fat thighs, and you perceive that your ideal self should have thin thighs, your specific self-esteem in that area might be low. If that becomes your focus, then your overall or global self-esteem might be low as well.

However, if your focus is on an internal quality, such as being an honest or caring person, your global self-esteem can be high even when your specific self-esteem is low in one area due, say, to perceived fat thighs. It is okay to identify and desire change in certain areas of your life. But it is important to keep those areas in perspective, and not make them the global or overall focus of who you are.

Take a minute or two each day to focus on yourself and all of the important, internal, unchanging qualities that comprise who you are. Think about the parts of you that you desire to modify or change. Set goals in those areas. Then make a plan to achieve those goals. This exercise is especially important for new mothers. Having a baby impacts every aspect of who you are. Sometimes, new mothers become so consumed with caring for the baby that they "lose sight" of themselves as individuals. They might begin to define themselves only as mothers, and forget to focus on the many other aspects of who they are.

For instance, let's say you are a wife, a daughter, a sister, and a friend. You might be loving, caring, giving, compassionate, loyal, dedicated, faithful, and kind. You are good at some things (list those things), and not so good at others (list those, too). Your hair is a certain color, and you have an appearance which is unique. List all the things you can think of about yourself.

Everyone occasionally feels inadequate and uncertain in some area. Maybe you feel inadequate as a mother because the baby is fussy today. When you have a balanced view of yourself, and all the many dimensions of your personality, you will gain confidence in those areas where you feel less competent. There is nothing healthy about always feeling worthless. Such feelings usually arise because you have made one specific area of your self-concept—an area in which you don't measure up to what you consider ideal—the primary focus.

Use the following exercise (the self-concept wheel) to prioritize the components of your self-concept. In doing this, refer back to the worksheets entitled Positive Things About Me, Me I Wish To Be, and Me I See. Then begin to focus on the internal, unchanging aspects of yourself that make you feel good. Prioritize those things.

Practice focusing on those positive things when you think about yourself. Place a lower priority on things that you would like to change, and then set your goals. If something cannot be changed, accept it and place the lowest priority on that aspect of you. Remember, you can change how you think about yourself. Positive self-esteem will help you have more confidence and be more successful at reaching your goals.

GETTING TO KNOW YOURSELF

Your Self-Concept Wheel

TAKE AN OPPORTUNITY to get to know yourself better. Few ever take the time to understand, let alone prioritize, the many components that make up their whole person. Doing so enhances your self-esteem, because it helps you to focus on your positive attributes, and to minimize and/or improve things you don't like.

Here's how the self-concept wheel works: You should have already listed many aspects of your self-concept on the previous pages in this book. Now, out of all those aspects, think of the three core components that help make up you. List those three in the center of the wheel. Next, in the second ring of the circle, list the next four most important aspects of your self-concept. In the third ring, list five more qualities or gifts that you have. Finally, in the outer ring, list four things about yourself that you would like to change or improve. Then you can use

Self-Concept Wheel

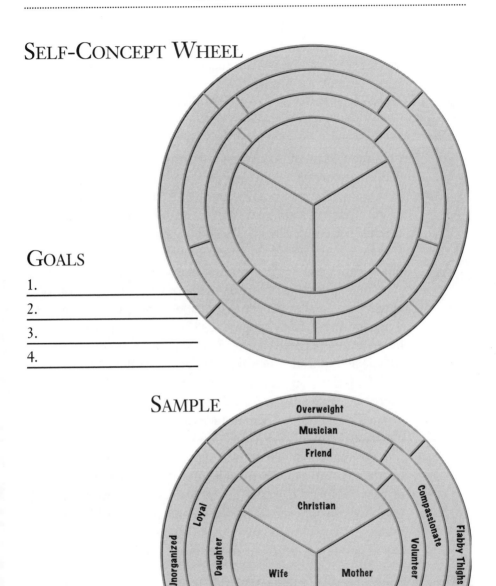

Goals

1. _____
2. _____
3. _____
4. _____

Sample

Goals

1. lose excess fat
2. tone my body
3. learn effective stress management
4. learn new organizational skills

these four items to help you set goals for self-improvement. A sample self-concept wheel is included for your use as a guide.

INTERNAL SOURCE OF CONTROL

DEVELOPING AN INTERNAL SOURCE of control is another important part of fostering a positive self-esteem. Internal source of control is a feeling that you have control over the events and circumstances in your life. That gives you a sense of power. External source of control, on the other hand, involves a feeling that events just happen to you at random, and you have very little control over the course of your life. It is a feeling that life controls you.

People with an internal source of control are action-oriented, because they believe that their actions make a difference. They are more likely to practice health-enhancing behaviors, because they believe that they have the power to improve their lives. Their attitude might be, "If I eat a healthy diet and exercise, I will live longer than if I don't." Those with an external source of control feel helpless and are less likely to take action on their own behalf. Their attitudes might be, "I'll die when I'm meant to die no matter what I do."

Teaching individuals to develop new coping skills increases internal source of control. The more power one feels over his or her own life, the greater that person's self esteem. If you feel you have control over your life, you are empowered to take the necessary steps to improve areas that need improving. That makes you feel good about yourself and it reduces stress.

POSITIVE BODY IMAGE

ENHANCING YOUR BODY IMAGE is a critical step in improving self-esteem and managing stress. Body image involves an inner view of the outer self which is created by your imagination. How you see your body, what you think about it, how you feel about it, how you experience it in motion, how you have perceived your body in the past, and what others have expressed to you in the past determine your body image today. You put all these things together in your imagination and formulate your ideas about your body. Body image is an evaluation of the physical self as a distinct object. It is impossible to separate body image and self-esteem, because body image is the most sensed part of the self.

Your body appearance is the only tangible aspect of your self. It is the part of you that you can see and touch, and the part which is seen and responded to by others. We all know there is much more to a person than his or her physical self and that individuals should not be judged only on appearance.

Yet in reality, physical appearance is a major factor in determining how we feel about ourselves and how others respond to us, and that makes it an important consideration for enhancing self-esteem and reducing stress. If you don't believe this, go to the store one day wearing no makeup, unkempt hair, tacky old clothes, and see how much confidence you have as you interact with others. Everyone can and should take positive steps to enhance body image and appearance, and improve health.

The first thing we recommend is for you to assess your current body image, appearance, and health status. If you have already completed the self-concept exercises, you have taken the first step to identifying positive things about yourself, as well as things that need improving. Second, take responsibility for making the changes you think you need. Remember, you alone are responsible. No one can do it for you. Third, commit yourself to taking action in these four areas:

- Exercise consistently.

- Eat a high-quality, low-fat diet.

- Practice effective stress-management strategies.

- Use cosmetics and clothes to your advantage.

■ STRIVING TOWARD GOALS

ANOTHER WAY TO MANAGE STRESS and enhance your self-esteem is to set goals, such as the ones you will set with the Body Contouring Program, and work toward achieving them. Setting and achieving realistic goals helps you recognize accomplishments, identify your skills and strengths, and feel responsible and capable. It helps you sort through your thoughts and your desires, and make realistic plans to achieve the things you want. We will discuss more about goal setting in the following chapters.

■ POSITIVE THINKING

POSITIVE SELF-TALK is a highly effective way to foster positive self-esteem and reduce stress. Your thoughts determine your attitude. You think, or talk to yourself mentally throughout the day. Often we are not even aware that we are talking to ourselves constantly. It is this self-talk that can make you your own best friend or your own worst enemy.

We cause a great deal of our own stress through how we think. The ability to control our thoughts and emotions requires effort and self-discipline, especially after having a baby. Remember, the hormonal changes combined with the extra responsibility and fatigue that come with having a new baby make us very vulnerable to negative thinking. We have to work harder during the postpartum period at controlling how we think. If you fail to exercise this control, postpartum adjustment will be more difficult. Your thinking or self-talk affects the way you feel, and how you feel will affect your ability to accomplish your goals.

Psychologists have identified several irrational thoughts that have been shown to cause stress for people in general. In my experience working with women who have had babies, I have found that they are more likely to think irrationally during the postpartum period. It is helpful to become familiar with common irrational thoughts, because once you understand what they are, and that they promote negative feelings, you can recognize them when they creep into your mind. Learn to substitute irrational thoughts with rational ones.

Following is a list of the most common irrational thoughts adapted from the work of Dr. Albert Ellis, founder of a form of counseling called Rational Emotive Therapy, to apply to postpartum women.[6] In 1961, Dr. Ellis began to teach people how to reduce stress. His solution was predicated on the avoidance of stressful or irrational thinking. By exposing self-defeating thought processes, Ellis's Rational Emotive Therapy states that you can retrain yourself to think in more productive ways. We have found his ideas to be very useful in working with postpartum women.

IRRATIONAL IDEAS

1. "Life should be fair."

2. "Everyone must like me and approve of me all the time."

3. "I must be perfect."

4. "My worth as a person depends on what I achieve or how I look."

5. "Other people cause my stress."

6. "I need someone else to make me happy."

7. "It's easier to avoid difficult situations than to face them."

8. "My way of looking at the world is the only way."

9. "I view things as awful or horrible when I get frustrated."

---

[6]Albert Ellis and Robert A. Harper, *A Guide to Rational Living* (Prentice-Hall: Englewood Cliffs, New Jersey, 1961)

10. "I have no control over what I think about or how I feel."

The following are more detailed explanations of the ten irrational ideas listed above, as well as suggestions for alternative ways of thinking which reduce stress.

RATIONAL OR PRODUCTIVE THINKING

1 Most of us grow up with the idea that life should be fair. Therefore, if things don't go the way we believe they should have gone, we become very upset. Maybe you expected to have a vaginal delivery—like your friend. But it turns out that you experienced complications and must have a cesarean. You might think, "It's not fair." Every time you think about your delivery in this way, you'll have a stress response. The fact is that life is not fair. We are going to have our share of frustration or unfairness. It is helpful to acknowledge that this is just the way life is, instead of dwelling on how it "should be." When you think this way, you can just brush off most seemingly unfair events as part of life, and move on.

2 You do not need to have approval from everyone, even all the people who are important to you, in order to be happy. Many of the things you do as a mother might be different from the way your mother, or your mother-in-law, thinks you should do them. To desire everyone's approval is an unattainable goal. The greater our need for approval, the less likely we are to get it. That is because if you are willing to do almost anything for the approval of others, you probably do not have a strong sense of your own identity and your own set of standards. You are probably too focused on what you can get from others, in the form of approval or affection, instead of what you can give.

Instead of striving to please others, your stress will be reduced if you work at loving and approving of yourself. By loving and accepting yourself and developing your own identity, you automatically become more appealing to others, without trying. Your focus is taken off of yourself, and is extended to others. You are better equipped to give approval and affection to others, instead of needing it from them. It is much like the old story of the cat determined to catch her tail. She ran around in circles as fast as she could chasing her tail—to no avail. The harder she chased, the farther it was from her grasp. It wasn't until she stopped chasing that the tail she desired fell within her reach.

3 You probably will not be instantly successful in everything you do. And that is okay because your value as a person does not depend on your accomplishments or failures. You might not be able to be superwoman and be the very best at everything. Achievement does not determine your worth. I believe that you have value because you were created in God's image. Your worth comes from accepting and knowing Him. Remind yourself to place emphasis on the actual participation in events or things— not on the outcome. Perfectionist thinking often causes fear of failure. In reality, success lies in playing the game, not in winning or losing.

4 Society wants you to believe that external things are the most important. Subsequently, advertisers make you feel deficient in all areas of your appearance and therefore entice you to purchase their products (with the hope of improvement). But you must remind yourself that external things, such as skin, hair, and fingernails are not the most important determinants of who you are. There is much more to you than your external package. To focus only on the outside would be as ridiculous as throwing out the contents of your microwave dinner, and eating the wrapper.

5 You are responsible for your own life and happiness. You can't place that burden on anyone else. You can choose to be angry or upset or even depressed, and you can choose to blame others. Blaming others is not the choice you want to make, because that can cause many emotional problems. Blaming is nonproductive, and it confuses the action with the person. Most people do the best they can with the resources available to them. Besides, we know that it is not our role to judge others for not behaving according to our specifications. If "to err is human," then I know that "forgiveness is sanity"—so I have a policy to forgive others and to forgive myself.

6 You know there is no such thing as a perfect human love relationship—except in fairy tales. Other people might look like they have a perfect relationship, because you only see them in public. But all successful relationships require commitment and hard work.

7 It is much easier to face difficult situations as they arise. If you avoid them, you will dwell on the problem anyway, and that will cause a great deal of stress. Things usually seem much worse than they actually turn out to be. So if you face the situation honestly and openly now, you will not fear the future and instead will gain self-respect and confidence.

8 Your perceptions are different from anyone else's. Other people have had unique experiences and might see the same event very differently. Remain open to the opinions of others.

9 Small children view things as "awful" when they become frustrated. Children cannot tolerate frustration, because they do not have the ability to think abstractly. They feel as though a particular moment of frustration will last forever, because they cannot project an end to it. As an adult, you can tolerate frustration because you have the ability to think beyond the frustration of the moment. If you acknowledge your frustration and begin to take action, you can remedy the situation. But if you "awful-ize" things, you become incapacitated and hinder yourself from seeking solutions.

10 You have control over what you think about and how you feel—for the most part. If you indulge yourself in thinking negatively, you will feel bad. But you can replace your negative thoughts with positive thoughts and as a result, you will feel positive.

POSITIVE AFFIRMATIONS

POSITIVE AFFIRMATIONS ALSO are valuable stress management tools. It would be nice to hear affirmations regarding the positive aspects of yourself from others, but sometimes you don't. However, there is someone whose voice you can always hear that can consistently provide you with positive affirmations—and that person is the one looking back when you look in the mirror.

Affirmations are positive statements about ourselves and our goals that we focus on every day. It is helpful to write your own list of affirmations and place it on your bathroom mirror, above your baby's changing table, or at least someplace where you will see it many times throughout the day. Every time you see the affirmations, repeat them several times in your head. Before you know it, you will develop a habit of thinking positively instead of negatively. It takes about six weeks to form the habit of thinking positively. The following are some examples of positive affirmations which will help you form the habit of positive thinking:

- "I love and accept myself as I am."

- "I was divinely created and have significance based on my relationship with Christ."

- "I have special talents and gifts, and a place in this world only I can fill."

- "I appreciate every moment of my life. I do not dwell on a dead past or an imagined future."

■ "I'm gentle, forgiving, and kind to myself and to others."

■ "I'm eager to accept new challenges, knowing that new experiences will help me grow."

■ "I love to take healthy risks, because I know that in order to feel, learn, change, grow, love, and live I must take many risks. The person who risks nothing, does nothing. The greatest risk is to risk nothing at all."

■ "I'm making daily progress in reaching my health and appearance goals."

Your desire to improve your appearance or your health is really your "thought" to improve. Any action you take had to be a thought first. Your attitudes about life are really nothing more than your consistent thoughts about life. Your entire future will be determined largely by your thoughts. Your determination to succeed is nothing more than your thoughts about success, which lead to feelings and actions that will make those thoughts reality.

Many of the most respected leaders focused on the power of thought, their minds, in determining how well their lives would go.

Ralph Waldo Emerson stated, "We become what we think about all day long."

Abraham Lincoln said, "People are about as happy as they make up their mind to be."

Norman Vincent Peale explained, "Change your thoughts and you change your world."

Even the Bible instructs us regarding our thoughts in the following passage: "Finally, brethren, whatever is true, whatever is honorable, whatever is just, whatever is pure, whatever is lovely, whatever is gracious, if there is any excellence, if there is anything worthy of praise, think about these things." (Philippians 4:8)

Think about it. You are responsible for what you think about. Once you learn to take control of your thoughts and to focus on the positive, becoming successful at reaching your goals in life will seem almost effortless—a natural progression of your thoughts.

VISUALIZING POSITIVE OUTCOMES

VISUALIZATION IS ANOTHER IMPORTANT SKILL in reducing stress and in reaching your goals. Not only is it important to think about what you want, but you should picture it as well. For example, instead of focusing on how out of shape you are after the birth of a baby, and how flabby your abdomen is, think about what a miraculous accomplishment your body has just performed. Now that your body has successfully accomplished that goal, you focus on images of your body as shapely and well toned.

Positive thoughts are your first step. Your mind stores away this image and begins to help you take steps daily that lead you closer to accomplishing this new goal. Remember, thoughts and images lead to actions. Imagine yourself already looking like what you consider ideal. It might help you to focus on an old picture of yourself before childbirth (if that is your "ideal") or to find a picture of someone who can be your role model.

CREATING A POSITIVE STATE OF MIND

ONE OF THE MOST IMPORTANT COMPONENTS of reducing stress and enhancing self-esteem is an understanding of how important it is for you to develop the habit of controlling your thoughts. We've all heard of the concept called "state of mind." You've heard people say, "He was in a bad state of mind when he failed the test," or "Happiness is a state of mind."

What do we mean when we talk about state of mind? Your state of mind is determined by a combination of mental and physiological processes. Mental processes include how positively or negatively you are thinking. Physical processes include your degree of muscular tension or relaxation, breathing rate and depth, blood pressure, heart rate, and other factors.

If you think about something stressful or negative, your body will respond by becoming tense and uptight, and you will be in a negative state. That is why we say you create how you feel. If a director of a movie wants you to feel scared, he creates and manipulates what you see and hear. He can produce a comedy or a tragedy out of the same event, depending on what he decides to put on the screen and how he presents it. Dramatic, frightening music causes you to tense up and expect something negative and places you in a negative state. You can do the same thing to yourself with your thoughts.

Worry, which is the expectation of something negative in the future, causes the same negative state of mind that the movie director created. Once you are in a negative state, the resources or options for behavior are mostly negative. Let's illustrate how this works. What if a friend was supposed to meet you for lunch at noon? You arrive ten minutes early, and at 12:30 P.M. your friend has still not arrived.

At this point, how you think about what is happening will determine your state and your behavior. You could assume or think that she forgot about the appointment. If you do, you automatically begin to tense your muscles, and your heart rate and breathing rate will increase. Your blood pressure will rise and certain chemical changes will take place in your body. This is a stress response. Your mind and your body have worked together to draw you into a negative state. Any action taken from this state will be negative.

*R*emember, negative states begin like small flames on a match. If allowed to burn, they catch on and explode into a flaming inferno.

Let's look at a different scenario. What if you had imagined your friend's tardiness as something you do not understand, but with the positive thoughts that something important must be happening in her life to prevent her from making your appointment? This time, your body remains relaxed and calm. Your state is positive. No matter what you find out later, you have been spared a costly detour into negativity. If nothing else, you might have just learned that this person is not reliable.

Remember, negative states begin like small flames on a match. If allowed to burn, they catch on and explode into a flaming inferno. You can snuff out a match flame with the touch of your fingers or a puff of air. But an inferno requires hours or even days to extinguish. And even when it is under control, there are damages that remain.

BECOMING MORE ASSERTIVE

ANOTHER IMPORTANT COPING STRATEGY for optimal mental health is assertiveness, which is not to be confused with passiveness or aggressiveness. Passiveness involves giving in to another's demands regardless of how it affects you. Aggressiveness is attempting to force your desires on others without consideration of their rights, needs, or desires. Assertiveness is respecting the rights and feelings of others, while expecting others to respect your rights and your feelings. The following is a comparison of passive, aggressive, and assertive individuals:

Sally is passive. She avoids expressing to others what she wants, thinks, or feels. If she does express herself, she speaks in ways which put her down. Apologetic words are often spoken, and she is silent much of the time. She allows others to make choices for her, and has difficulty deciding something as simple as what restaurant she would like to go to for dinner. You often hear Sally saying such things as, "I'm sorry"; "you know"; "I mean"; "I guess." She might pout or sulk instead of confronting you if you hurt her feelings, and she hopes you will guess or figure out what's wrong. Her voice is weak, hesitant, and soft. Her eyes are downcast, and she agrees with everything others say.

Sara is aggressive. She says what she wants, thinks, and feels no matter what, even if it is at the expense of others, and she believes her way is the only way of doing things. She uses loaded words and statements directed at others which label them or cast blame, instead of using "I" statements and expressing things in terms of how it makes her feel. She threatens and accuses, and consistently interrupts others when they try to express their point of view. She has an air of superiority about her, and usually appears tense and angry. It might seem as though she has a "chip on her shoulder," or that she thinks the world "owes her something."

Sue is assertive. She says what she honestly wants, thinks, and feels in direct, helpful and consistent ways. She makes her own choices and communicates using "I" statements, which indicate how she feels without judging the feelings of others. She is able to listen to others and she communicates caring and strength. Her voice is firm, warm, and sincere, and she makes eye contact when she speaks. She is able to express her needs while taking into consideration the needs of others.

Being assertive means that you recognize your rights and the rights of others. One of the most important times for you to utilize assertive behavior is after the birth of your baby. You must assert yourself in asking for help and emotional support from those around you, while understanding (if they are family members) that they might be experiencing additional stress, too.

One of the most important times for you to utilize assertive behavior is after the birth of your baby. You must assert yourself in asking for help and emotional support from those around you.

Still, you need help caring for the baby so that you can take time for yourself each day. That time alone allows you to maintain balance in your life and not become consumed by motherhood. That might mean your husband or another support person needs to find forty-five minutes in his or her schedule to watch the new baby (and other siblings), so that you can get out and exercise, or spend time alone in relaxation, napping, or some other self-care activity. This time to yourself is essential in your recovery and it will make your mothering tasks much more enjoyable. Here are some tips on asserting yourself in making daily private time a priority:

■ Convince yourself that you deserve free time to do whatever you want, whether that involves exercising, thinking, or something else. Realize that without self-care time, it is difficult to maintain emotional energy, patience and perspective—three of the ingredients essential to motherhood.

■ Be consistent in requesting that others leave you alone and not intrude on your private time.

■ Make arrangements with your partner so that he truly understands your need to have him take over your responsibilities during this time—consistently—so that you can be the best possible wife and mother.

■ If chores must be left undone in order for you to have your private time, leave the chores. Your time alone is more important. Your mental and physical health is worth a lot more than a clean kitchen!

■ Make sure your daily private time is a time free of responsibility. You need a mental break from the constant burden of being the person in charge of the safety and well-being of your new baby (and other children).

In order to maximize enjoyment of your private time, you need to let go of guilty feelings about not doing certain household chores. You can't be the best at everything, and some things have to slide. Remember, don't let the thing that slides be your mental well-being.

Following are some tips that will help you become more assertive. If you can learn to be assertive in some areas of your life, the skill will likely transfer into other areas as well.

■ **Compliment others.**
Practice giving others sincere compliments. Many unassertive people hesitate to give compliments, because they feel others would not value what they have to say. Giving compliments reinforces you that people do care what you think and say.

■ **Use "I" statements.**

Many unassertive people are hesitant to use the word "I" because it implies ownership, and disagreement with an "I" statement by someone else is often seen as rejection by the unassertive person. Don't be afraid to take a position. Let your preferences be known, because if you don't they will never be realized.

■ **Initiate conversation with others.**

Many unassertive people are too shy to initiate conversation with anyone who is not a close friend. Volunteer to be a greeter at church or at a social event. It builds confidence to learn to assert yourself in interactions with others. Plus, it feels good to other people for someone to take the time and energy to greet them.

■ **Ask "Why?"**

For unassertive people, it is often difficult to ask why—for fear that it represents a challenge to others. But asking "why" simply indicates you would like to have additional information. In many cases it is very appropriate. Ask your doctor why certain things were done. You have the right to know, and you have a need to understand.

■ **Use eye contact.**

This is the most difficult thing for the unassertive person to do. Whatever you do, don't look down when you are speaking or listening to someone else. That doesn't mean you have to stare at them. But maintain gentle eye contact, and show through your expression and attention that you value what the other person is saying.

■ **Say "No."**

When someone asks you to do something you cannot or do not wish to do, say no right then. Many nonassertive people will give an evasive response such as "Maybe" or "I'll let you know," when the real answer is "No."

Saying no at the time will allow the other person to make alternate plans, and will prevent you from having to worry about turning them down later, after they've had their hopes up. This will help you gain more self-respect, because you will be interacting with others honestly and assertively.

Becoming more assertive is a habit. You will notice that the more assertive you become, the more self-confidence and self-respect you will feel. Assertiveness boosts self-esteem.

TIME MANAGEMENT

OFTEN, it might seem that the clock is against you. But time moves at a predetermined rate, and we all have the same amount of it. Time can be on your side if you organize your life to use it to your benefit. The use of time is an endless series of management decisions. Inappropriate decisions might lead to frustrations, lower self-esteem, and increased stress. The important thing is to learn to plan your time so that you are able to do the things that you want to do. When you do waste time, waste it doing things that you consider fun and pleasurable.

Here is a list of common time-wasters which often go unnoticed, but might keep you from doing the things you enjoy:

■ **Disorganization.**
This is a key time-waster. If considerable time is spent searching for misplaced items, you might want to consider organizing for more efficient time usage.

■ **Procrastination.**
Putting things off usually costs us time in the long run, because we waste time thinking about whatever it is that we have failed to do. Putting off or delaying work is often caused by setting impossibly high standards. If you believe the task simply cannot be done, you probably attempt to ignore the work or put it off indefinitely.

Another problem is in looking at a project and feeling overwhelmed. When we do this, we don't know where to begin. Break projects down into small segments, and do those one at a time.

■ **Inability to say no.**
When you take on more than you can handle, your quality time and your health suffer. Saying no does not need to offend, and it is much more effective than saying yes, only to have to cancel at the last minute. Know your limitations.

■ **Visitors.**
Controlling time taken up by visitors requires courtesy and judgment. Prearrange times that you will allow visitors and discourage people from dropping in on you unannounced.

■ **Telephone calls.**
The telephone can be a constant interruption if you let it. Screen your calls with an answering machine during times when you are doing other things, or take it off the hook. Do not allow your relaxation time to be interrupted by the telephone.

■ **Watching television.**
Often it is tempting to leave the television set on all day, even if there's nothing on that you want to watch. The problem with this is that you might end up wasting time watching something that you really didn't intend to watch—simply because it's there. Instead, you will save time if you decide in advance which programs to watch, tape those programs using your VCR, and then watch them when they fit into your schedule. The rest of the time, leave the TV set off!

There are many time-savers which are important to utilize:[7]

- **Make use of services.**
  If cleaning house is something you do not want to spend your time doing, hire someone to help you. This will allow you to spend more time doing those things you consider most important.

- **Learn to double up on time.**
  Exercise while you watch television, cook while listening to music or talking on the phone, etc.

- **Utilize small segments of time.**
  Make a grocery list while heating baby bottles. Plan small projects while you wait for an appointment.

- **Plan ahead.**
  Prepare your "to-do" list for the next day each evening. If there are small tasks you can do in the evening to get a head start on the next day, such as setting out tomorrow's clothes or sterilizing bottles, do them.

RELAXATION

EVERYONE NEEDS TIME TO RELAX. Relaxation is a very important coping skill, and it involves more than distraction. Relaxation is a physical response that is the opposite of the stress response. Note the way your body feels when you're under stress. You discover that you tense your muscles in certain parts of your body. Some of us get a stiff neck, or tight shoulders, or a sore back. You might even clench your jaw and grit your teeth, which often causes headaches. You might even be so stressed so much of the time that the tension in your muscles becomes the norm. You can actually forget how to relax your muscles.

The stress response is the physiological change that takes place in your body when you experience stress. It is often called

[7]S. Winston, *Getting Organized*. (Warner Books: New York. 1978)

the fight-or-flight response, because our gut instinct is usually to fight someone, or to run away. Most of the time you don't act on this instinct, but the feeling is there. This stress response includes: increased muscle tension, increased heart rate, increased blood pressure, increased breathing rate, increased acid in the stomach, and other changes. Fight-or-flight becomes a major health hazard when fired too often or for too long. An estimated 50 to 80 percent of all diseases in this country have stress-related origins.

Like stress, relaxation changes our physiology, but in the opposite way. Relaxation reduces muscle tension, lowers heart rate, lowers blood pressure, reduces breathing rate, and increases the ability of the immune system to function. Experiencing true relaxation is like hitting a reset button.

There are many ways to relax. One is to use mental imagery, or visualization. Sit down in a comfortable, quiet spot where you will not be disturbed. Visualize yourself in a setting that you find relaxing. Maybe it is a sandy beach or a mountain peak. Focus your thoughts on this relaxing place and on what it feels like to be there. What are the sounds you hear in this relaxing place? Maybe you hear the birds chirping or the waves rolling into the shore. Be sure to take deep breaths and to let go of any tension you might be feeling in your body. Can you see the seagulls, or leaves dancing in the breeze?

The more you can involve your senses, the more you will be able to relax. What can you feel? Perhaps you feel the warmth of the sun beaming down on your skin. Maybe you feel the coolness of a mountain breeze caressing your face. Maybe you smell the scent of wildflowers or green grass, or taste the salt in the ocean air. Whatever place you are imagining, visualize as much detail as you can. Your body responds to this imaginary place in the same way as if it were real, so you will get a physiological relaxation response much the same as if you were really there, experiencing this place.

Doing this type of relaxation even for five or ten minutes will help you hit a reset button and will give you a sense of well-being and energy that you never dreamed possible. Being able to visualize for relaxation is a skill, and it requires some practice. It might take longer for you at first to learn to focus your thoughts and to avoid letting distracting thoughts creep in. With time, you will become very good at visualization. When you do, you will realize that it can help you in every area of your life.

One of the most important skills I used to get through my doctoral program was visualization. Not only did it allow me to relax when I needed to, but it also allowed me to build confidence. Before I would take an exam, or do an oral presentation (such as a doctoral defense, where you must meet with five or six professors and orally defend your dissertation to their satisfaction) I would visualize myself going through the experience perfectly. I would picture what I was saying, and my committee members responding positively. I would visualize taking my exam, feeling calm and enjoying the process of demonstrating what I had learned. By the time the actual event came up, I felt like I had already done it several times and been successful. So in a way, I knew what to expect and I knew I would be successful. This works for Body Contouring as well. It is very helpful to visualize yourself looking and feeling great, and to visualize your body enjoying walking, eating healthy, and feeling great.

■ ■ ■ ■ ■ ■ ■
*P*rogressive relaxation is helpful because it can be done almost any time to relieve tension.

Another type of relaxation is called progressive relaxation, which involves a tensing and relaxing of different muscle groups. Progressive relaxation is helpful because it can be done almost any time to relieve tension. One way to do this is to begin with your head, and work your way down your body. Start with the muscles in your face. Shut your eyes tightly and furrow your brow, and hold for about three seconds. Release all the muscles in your forehead and around your eyes. Take a mental note of the difference between tension in those muscles, and relaxation.

Next, wrinkle your nose and squeeze the muscles in your jaw and mouth area; hold for three seconds, and release. Then tense the muscles in your neck; hold, and release. Progress to your shoulders, arms, hands, chest, abdomen, buttocks, thighs, calves, feet, and finally, toes. When you have gone through each muscle group as described, you should be left feeling relaxed. If you practice this exercise regularly, you will actually be teaching your body and your mind what it means to be relaxed. With time, you will simply be able to think, "I need to relax," and your body will automatically begin to relax as if you had gone through a progressive relaxation session.

EXERCISE

ONE OF THE MOST BENEFICIAL COPING STRATEGIES you can use during the postpartum period is aerobic exercise. That is because exercise is beneficial to your mental and physical health. Mentally, the type of exercise recommended in our program is beneficial because it requires you to take time out for yourself several days each week. It gets you out of your routine and helps free your mind from the tensions of the day.

Low-intensity aerobic exercise has a therapeutic, clearing effect on your mind. Some people say this is due to the rhythm of walking. This type of exercise also releases endorphins, which are natural pain killers in the body. Endorphins have been shown to elevate mood for several hours after you exercise. We've all heard of a "runner's high." Low intensity exercise actually makes us feel "high." And the positive effects of exercise are not limited to the duration of your activity, but extend well beyond it. Aerobic exercise also automatically causes you to practice deep breathing, which enhances relaxation.

The Body Contouring Program is designed to help you improve health, lose weight, and tone your muscles. You will actually set goals and reach them. As you begin to experience success, you will be motivated to continue until you reach your goals. Exercise improves your ability to handle stress, and minimizes your chances of experiencing postpartum blues and long-term stress. You will know exactly what you need to do and the results you can expect. It has been specifically designed to help postpartum women regain shape and optimize health by experts in fitness and exercise physiology, health science, and obstetrics and gynecology.

CHAPTER NINE

Regaining Control of Your Life

"I t was 7:30 in the morning," Vicki said during a postpartum session. "My husband was ready for work, and he looked sharp. His clothes were pressed and starched, and he was alert, bright-eyed, and ready to face the world. He seemed so together, and I became angry as I watched him."

"What's the matter?" her husband asked.

"I don't know," she replied.

"It just bothered me to look at him, and then to look at myself. I was still in my robe, hadn't even been able to think about taking a shower yet, was drowsy and fatigued from being up in the night, and was aware that I would probably be in about the same condition at noon. It had been a long time since I had worn crisp, freshly starched clothing. My life was so disorganized. Time had lost all meaning. Some days it would be 6:00 in the evening and Hank would come home from work.

" 'What did you do today?' he would ask. And I would try to think of something significant to say. 'What did I do today?' I'd ask myself. 'Let's see, I changed three dirty diapers,' ...and other than that, it was difficult to recall. Yet I knew I had been busy all day. Things just seemed chaotic, and I was in a rut!"

As Vicki shared her story, I couldn't help thinking how typical it was. Having a baby can leave us feeling out of control. It becomes difficult to follow a regular routine, and with our schedules constantly changing, things seem chaotic and stressful. It is not uncommon for us to feel threatened as our husbands dress up and head out into the work world, while we're left feeling unattractive and isolated at home. During this time, we might envy and even resent our husband's freedom, and we might feel trapped and disorganized.

We've already discussed many of the most effective coping strategies for managing stress. Now we're going to focus on organizing our lives so that we feel a greater sense of control and effectiveness, and so that we have plenty of time in our schedules to devote to exercise and relaxation.

PLANNING THE DAY WITH BABY

PRODUCTIVE PLANNING is a critical factor in achieving the goals you set for yourself and your family—especially after you have a baby. If you constantly suffer through periods of not knowing where your time went, or not getting the most important things done, take this opportunity to rethink your planning skills. There are three tools we believe to be essential for effective daily planning with your new baby—a day-by-day appointment calendar; a small, purse-size notebook; and a daily to-do list.

The calendar is where you write down important events and appointments that you might make days, weeks, or even months in advance. Each morning as you make out your to-do list for that day, take a look at your calendar and see if anything from the calendar needs to be included on your to-do list. For example, if you notice you have a doctor's appointment in two days, it will be marked on your calendar. Your to-do list for that day will need to include arranging a babysitter for your appointment. The small notebook is where you jot down errands and other tasks as they occur to you. You keep this notebook with you, in your purse or pocket all the time.

Your daily to-do list can be written on a page in your notebook. It is compiled first thing in the morning for that day, and it includes each of the things you intend to do during the course of the day. It might be helpful to prioritize each item on your list, from most important to least. This will help you make sure you get the items you consider essential done. If everything you intend to do one day does not get done, jot down the unfinished items in your notebook and include them in your list for the following day, or delete them. Include your daily exercise session as one of the top priorities on your to-do list.

There are several reasons a system, such as the one we've just described, becomes essential after having a baby. Caring for an infant and/or small children requires so much thought and focus that it is difficult to hold anything else in your mind for any length of time. Before I had a baby, my friend Cindy told me that since her two-year-old daughter had been born, she had lost many brain cells. I asked her what she meant, and she said that after her daughter was born, she was unable to remember anything, or to be effective at getting things done. She explained that many times she would find herself driving in the car and she wouldn't even remember what errand she was supposed to be running. She said that she would be walking through the mall and would not remember what she came for, or she would come home from the grocery store without many of the items she planned to purchase.

If everything you intend to do one day does not get done, jot down the unfinished items in your notebook and include them in your list for the following day, or delete them.

"She is just scatterbrained," I thought to myself as I listened to her problems. "Things would never be like that for me." I didn't appreciate the full extent of what she was describing until my son was born. Cindy's words came back to me when I found myself doing the same things. That was when I realized I must have a system. I also understood what was happening and why. It's not that you lose brain cells when you have a baby. Instead, we have a new responsibility that is so complex and so important, it demands the vast majority of our focus.

It's like working on a doctoral dissertation (only magnified about a million times in importance!). A counselor friend was working on his dissertation at the same time I was working on mine. One day he came to the offices of the medical clinic where we both worked, looking like he had seen a ghost. I asked him what was wrong, and he explained that he had forgotten to pick up his five-year-old daughter from preschool. It was his day to pick her up, as he did every week, and he didn't show up.

How could he have forgotten something so important? The answer is that no matter how smart we are, we can only store a certain amount of information in our brains at one time. He was at the library, focused upon the many complex issues of his dissertation, and he was unable to access any other information at the time. He needed a to-do list to trigger his memory. When your brain is occupied with the complex issues of being a mom, a to-do list helps you remember other things.

Here's how it works. Think of your brain as being like a closet. It will hold a great deal, but only a few things can be at the front of the closet. Some things have to be pushed to the back, and there comes a point when no more can be shoved in at all, or when you have to throw some things out to fit others in. When you have a baby, taking care of that baby (and other children if you have them) fills up most of the space in your "brain" closet. Everything else must be squeezed into the back, or might not fit in at all. That's why it becomes essential to write down any and everything you want to do—everything! Even though it might seem clear to you in the morning what errands you need to run that afternoon, or that you are supposed to go to a party that evening, you can be sure that something will happen with the baby and you will quickly shove everything else to the back.

One day when Michael was about six weeks old, I carefully strapped him into his car seat in the back seat of our car, and headed out to run errands. It was a peaceful day and I had a very clear picture in my mind of where I needed to go and what I needed to do. I was driving along a curvy road near our country home, headed towards town, and I glanced in my rearview mirror to check on my precious little companion. As I peered into the back seat, I saw nothing! There was no car seat and no baby. I can't tell you all of the things that flashed through my mind in that instant: "Someone has kidnapped my baby. I forgot to bring him. No, I'm positive I strapped him in. I'm losing my mind."

I quickly pulled over to the side of the road, jumped out of the front seat and opened the door to the back seat. There was

Michael in his car seat, flipped upside down on the left side of the back seat and just hanging there, wedged between the front and back seat—suspended a few inches above the floorboard. I turned the car seat over and he was smiling, completely unaware that anything was out of the ordinary. As I sat there and tried to catch my breath, things began to make sense. My husband had put the car seat in his car for a family outing the previous day. That morning, he told me he had put the car seat back in my car. I assumed he had strapped the car seat in, but he had just set it in its position in the middle of the back seat. So the baby was strapped into the car seat, but the car seat was not strapped into the car.

Needless to say, after this happened, I couldn't remember anything I was planning on doing that day. The moral of this story is the only thing you can expect once you have children is the unexpected. A to-do list would have quickly and easily cued me back into what I needed to do. Since that time, I rarely leave the house without checking the car seat, and making sure I have my list!

TAKING ADVANTAGE OF YOUR PEAK ENERGY HOURS

HAVE YOU EVER HEARD SOMEONE SAY "I am a morning person," or "I am a night person"? Most mothers who have newborns are forced to become both, although they have a natural tendency to function better at one time or the other. Most people, during the course of a day, go through regular cycles of energy. A typical schedule would be as follows:

8:00 A.M. TO 12:00 NOON	HIGH ENERGY LEVEL
12:00 P.M. TO 3:00 P.M.	MEDIUM ENERGY LEVEL
3:00 P.M. TO 6:00 P.M.	LOW ENERGY LEVEL
6:00 P.M. TO 9:00 P.M.	MEDIUM TO HIGH ENERGY LEVEL
AFTER 9:00 P.M.	RESTING OR VERY LOW ENERGY LEVEL

Most people operate on high energy the first few hours in a day and then drop until a late-afternoon low, when they feel like resting or napping. Energy levels often rise again in the early evening. This is a second high. Another evening drop after the second high leads to rest again and eventually to sleep. However, there are "night" people who have trouble adjusting to this type of schedule. They are more likely to have morning lows which perk up around noon and through late afternoon, decline after dinner, and surge again about 10:00 P.M. until past midnight.

Knowing your peak energy times will help you arrange your tasks around your own energy fluctuations. Try to arrange your to-do list, and possibly your newborn's schedule, around your energy levels. Your "high" hours would be the optimal time to exercise, perform tasks which require intense concentration or original thinking, or tasks which are unpleasant or stressful, or require a lot of motivation and energy. Don't put off exercise until a low-energy time, if you can help it. You will be more likely to remain consistent if you schedule your exercise session during a high energy time, and at the same time each day.

Reserve medium times for fairly routine work such as picking up the house or planning dinner, going to the grocery store, etc. During your low-energy hours, plan a nap for you and the baby; or if the baby is awake, use this time to play with him or her; write letters; read a magazine; talk on the phone; relax; watch television; read; etc.

If you must perform tasks which normally require high energy at one of your low-energy times, give yourself a lift with a high-energy snack—such as a small glass of juice or skim milk, a piece of fruit, a small piece of turkey or chicken, or some low-fat yogurt. Eating too much will cause you to quickly tire. One piece of fruit, one-half a serving of yogurt, or six to eight ounces of juice will be enough to give you an energy boost. Eat your snack about fifteen minutes before your task.

Blood-sugar levels are believed to be a factor in mood and energy levels. In other words, if your blood sugar is low, you will feel tired and possibly "blue" or down. You might need to boost your blood sugar level by eating a small snack. Eating too much will cause a quick surge in blood sugar levels followed by a big drop—and a subsequent drop in energy.

TIME-SAVING HOUSEKEEPING TIPS

MOST OF US require a certain degree of order in the home. It makes us feel as though we are in control of our lives, and being in control is important for stress management. The most effective and efficient time-saving housekeeping tip for the postpartum period is to hire a housekeeper. If you can afford to hire someone to come in once a week and do a thorough cleaning, it will save you several much-needed hours each week during which you can do other things (things which will help you recover and get back in shape). Perhaps your mother, sister, or a friend could help you if hiring a housekeeper is not an option. But if you don't have outside help, this section offers time-saving tips on keeping a moderately clean house. The time you save can be applied to exercise, relaxation, or other enjoyable activities.

If you have to do it yourself, try to make cleaning the house a form of exercise. Think of it as an activity which can help you burn more fat.

If you have to do it yourself, try to make cleaning the house a form of exercise. Think of it as an activity which can help you burn more fat. Cleaning house is like exercise, in that it might be one of the few things you do during a day which gives you a clear, tangible sense of accomplishment. The most important step in effective cleaning after having a baby is setting up a system that you follow consistently.

Allow yourself one hour and fifteen minutes per day, scheduled during your medium energy time, and divide this time as follows. (Remember, don't waste your high-energy times on housekeeping. Do this type of mindless task during medium or even low-energy times):

■ **Priority One.**
These are those jobs that must be performed daily.

Allow forty-five minutes for priority-one tasks, such as cleaning the kitchen, picking up clutter, taking out the garbage, etc.

■ **Priority Two.**

These are jobs that need to be done about twice per week. Allow thirty minutes per day on priority-two jobs—working on only as many as will fit in that time slot. These jobs might include laundry, changing the sheets, sweeping, vacuuming, and scouring bathrooms. You might want to pick one of these jobs per day to focus on.

■ **Priority Three.**

These are jobs that need to be done once a week or less. Set aside one extra one-hour session per week for priority-three jobs, such as mopping floors, and dusting and polishing furniture. If you do everything yourself and you follow this schedule, you will spend about an hour and fifteen minutes per day on the house, with one day being a long day (two hours and fifteen minutes).

Consider doing your housework while the baby is awake. Strap him or her in a front pack, and you'll both enjoy the closeness. Save the baby's nap time to take a nap yourself, or to do other things you can't do while he or she is awake. If you hire a person to clean once a week, instruct her to take care of priority-two and -three jobs, and as many of the priority-one jobs as she can get done.

This will free a great deal of time for you to spend in more productive ways. You will go from spending an hour and fifteen minutes daily, to about forty-five minutes daily or less, plus you will free up the one hour per week that you would spend on priority-three jobs. That means you would gain four-and-a-half hours per week.

If you don't hire a housekeeper, decide with your family which responsibilities will be dedicated to your husband or other members. Once an agreement is made, post a sign in the kitchen listing who is responsible for what. That way, there is no questioning who is accountable if the task is left undone. This posting of responsibilities also helps other members of the family see how many responsibilities you have, and why you cannot be expected to do everything. Otherwise, you might get taken for granted.

Kim came to my office shortly after her daughter was born, saying that she was completely overwhelmed at the number of responsibilities that fell on her shoulders every day. Before having a baby, she had worked and was in school. At that time, her husband John realized the need for them to share the household responsibilities. Kim explained that he often would cook dinner, clean up the kitchen, pitch in with the laundry, and just do his share.

"But he has totally changed since Taylor was born," Kim said. "I guess since I no longer leave the house each day to go to school or work, he feels that I have plenty of time to do everything around the house. This is very difficult for me, doing all the housework—even chores that he used to always do, plus taking care of a newborn baby and trying to allow time to get back in shape mentally and physically. Yet I feel guilty for needing more help because, after all, John is working and I'm 'just staying home.'"

Over time, Kim had become angrier and angrier at John for not helping, yet she felt guilty that she couldn't do it all. The "ideal" wife and mother could do it all—right?

"As hard as I try, things are left undone," Kim said. "There are many days when the only time I sit down is to breast-feed Taylor, and yet it still isn't enough."

Kim knew how important it was to take care of herself, and to allow personal time each day. (Don't fall into the trap of thinking this is a selfish way to think. Everyone in your family suffers if you don't allow yourself personal self-improvement time and quiet time.) But she explained that the only way she could do all the household chores was if she gave up her personal time.

We decided Kim needed to sit down and make a list of the things she was expected to do each day. She kept the list up for one week. At the end of the week, she was amazed at all the things she was responsible for. Her list for each day filled up two full legal pad sheets of paper. Looking at this list, she realized that things needed to change, and she need not feel guilty.

"It wasn't as if I had left my full-time career to become a full-time housekeeper," she said. "I had decided to stay home to become a full-time mommy. Taking care of an infant is a full-time job. Just because I'm staying home does not mean I suddenly have all the time in the world."

When Kim showed John her list of responsibilities, things began to change.

"I think this was the first time he really realized that I could not do it all and he needed to pitch in the way he used to," she said. "He had to see, on paper, how much I was doing in order to realize I still needed his help. So we divided household responsibilities and made out a list with our initials beside the chores that we would do. We posted the list on the refrigerator so there would be no mistaking who was supposed to do what."

■ ■ ■ ■ ■ ■
The most important step is to get into a system in which you can spend the least time possible on chores so that you will have time available to spend working toward your goals.

This type of objective system works quite well. Remember, taking care of a baby is a full-time job. Just because you are at home does not mean that you have a lot of free time on your hands. Everyone needs to pitch in with household responsibilities. Each task that you can delegate to someone else will free up valuable, personal time for you. The most important step is to get into a system in which you can spend the least time possible on chores so that you will have time available to spend working toward your goals. The cleanest and most organized house in the world will not make you happy if you are not happy with yourself. The most important thing you can do for yourself and for your family is to spend time each day working on maximizing your own health and appearance. Remember, your level of self-esteem is the most powerful determining factor for how you behave, how you treat others, and how you feel.

One of my clients, Sarah, had considered coming to talk to me several times. However, each time she would schedule an appointment, she would cancel at the last minute saying she could not afford to come in at that time. She was carrying around quite a bit of excess fat weight since her baby was born, and she went through phases of being very motivated to shape up. But when it came down to actually having to invest in this effort, her motivation was not there.

When Sarah finally hit rock bottom, feeling very blue, unattractive, and unhealthy, she made an appointment to come see me and kept it. As we began to discuss what she had been experiencing, she explained that every time she would feel down about her weight, she would decide to come in; but then she would start thinking about all the things she could buy with the money she would have to spend on the session. So she would cancel the appointment and go shopping. She had purchased several new outfits, a very expensive chair, and several other pieces of furniture as she attempted to avoid her real problem.

Sarah explained that each time she bought something, she would expect it to make her feel better, but instead she would become more depressed as she realized that these things she was buying really could not make her happy. She said that she would sit there, in the sharpest looking house in town, with the finest clothes money could buy, and cry because she felt so lacking.

After she finally made the decision to shape up, and had the willingness to do whatever it took, she began to get results. As her success progressed, she said she finally realized that as she became happy with herself, she began to understand how insignificant her material possessions were. There is little joy to be found in a chair or a blouse or a clean house, if you haven't taken care of yourself.

An old saying was posted over the door in the fitness room at a college where I used to teach. It said, "There once was a man who spent his health to gain his wealth, then turned around and spent all his wealth trying to regain his health." What matters are people—ourselves and others, and our most valuable time investments are the ones we make accordingly.

■ GOAL SETTING, MOTIVATION AND SUCCESS STRATEGIES

WHAT DO YOU THINK OF when you hear the word "success"? Ralph Waldo Emerson[8] described success in this way:

"To laugh often and much; to win the respect of intelligent people and the affection of children; to earn the appreciation of honest critics and endure the betrayal of false friends; to appreciate beauty; to find the best in others; to leave the world a bit better, whether by a healthy child, a garden patch or a redeemed social condition; to know even one life has breathed easier because you have lived. This is to have succeeded."

This is a profound and lovely definition of success. A person who lives in the manner described above is a person who has learned to take control of her own life and who is able to consistently set and strive toward personal goals. Success is actually a way of living, rather than a destination to be reached. It is the ongoing process of striving to learn and grow—to become more. It is a progressive course. The successful path involves defining your goals, taking action, reviewing the results you are getting, and having the flexibility to change or alter your course until you reach your goals. You must know what your goal or target is so that you can move toward it. Then you must gain information regarding the techniques to follow, or the steps to take in order to reach your goal.

■ ■ ■ ■ ■ ■
Take a few minutes to set some reasonable goals for the postpartum period. You might have three or five major goals. Your goals should be major accomplishments that you wish to make.

Take a few minutes to set some reasonable goals for the postpartum period. You might have three or five major goals.

---

[8]Caesar Johnson, *To See a World in a Grain of Sand* (C.R. Gibson Company: Norwalk, Connecticut, 1972)

Your goals should be major accomplishments that you wish to make. An example would be, "I will lose thirty pounds of excess fat on the Body Contouring Program."

Once you've set your major goals, outline the steps you must take to reach your goals. These steps are called objectives. Your objectives must be specific and measurable. You should be able to look back at the end of each week and determine whether or not you have met your objectives. Objectives for the goal listed above might be:

1 "I will follow the daily walking schedules in the Body Contouring Program for twelve weeks."

2 "I will avoid foods from the Five Fat Groups and will eat five to six healthy meals per day."

Next comes the most critical step—taking action. This is where many people fall short of reaching their goals. Knowledge of what you want, and information regarding how to get it, is useless unless we are willing to "do what it takes." If we want to have the power to change our lives, we must take action. In fact, the word power is defined as the "ability to act or produce an effect."

Once you begin to take action, you must evaluate the results you are getting, and be willing to make modifications— if necessary—regarding your course. The Body Contouring Program is designed to enable you to utilize these principles to set your life on the "success" course during the postpartum period.

Remember that as you pursue your goals there is no such thing as failure. There are only results from which you can learn. Many women have a strong fear of failure. This fear is actually a fear of being judged and found lacking. No one who expects to walk off with a "blue ribbon" or "first prize" is afraid of being judged. Those of us who respond poorly to failure do so because we have not grown to see failure as a necessary part of the learning process.

As a young girl, you might have been taught to be "sugar and spice." You might have been taught to view failure as something wrong or bad. It poses a threat to your receiving approval as a "good girl." Worrying about approval in this way is unproductive and inhibits action. It leads to procrastination. We might decide not to take action unless we are sure we cannot fail. This type of all-or-none thinking creates more problems.

Imagine giving your child a report card and accepting only a 100 as a passing grade. Anything below that is failure. So a grade of 98 percent is a failing grade. As unreasonable as this sounds, it is the type of system to which many of us hold ourselves accountable. It is a pass/fail system in which the requirements are so stringent that passing is nearly impossible. If you place a child on such a system, how long do you think it would take for him or her to cease to be motivated to try anything?

When you hold yourself to perfectionist standards, the outcome is avoidance. You might be avoiding failure by: 1) not trying; 2) limiting your investments; or 3) not finishing what you start. This way, if you do not get the outcome you desire, you can discredit your performance as not being a valid indicator of your ability because you didn't really try. The problem with this type of system is that it becomes impossible to ever achieve what you desire. Why? Because you never fully commit yourself to an endeavor.

It makes sense to commit to something only when you can trust yourself to hang in there when the going gets tough, and to give it all you've got. If you are always trying to protect yourself from the possibility of failure, you will be likely to quit when times are difficult. This tendency is often called "learned helplessness," which is the premature conclusion that one's attempts will not be good enough, and it disrupts behavior by undermining motivation. Learned helplessness destroys persistence. The moment you feel that success might be complicated, you're tempted to give up.

However, you can learn new and effective ways of viewing failure, which is really nothing more than feedback. Feedback tells you what works and what does not work. It tells you what to do next time and allows you to anticipate success in the future. Think about the man who:

failed in business at age thirty-one

was defeated in a legislative race at age thirty-two

failed again in business at age thirty-four

overcame the death of his sweetheart at age thirty-five

had a nervous breakdown at age thirty-six

lost an election at age thirty-eight

lost a congressional race at age forty-three

lost a congressional race at age forty-six

lost a congressional race at age forty-eight

lost a senatorial race at age fifty-five

failed in an effort to become vice-president at age fifty-six

lost a senatorial race at age fifty-eight

was elected President of the United States at age sixty

The man was Abraham Lincoln. Do you think he could have ever become president if he had allowed his failures to get him down?

And what about Thomas Edison? After he had made 9,999 attempts at perfecting the light bulb and hadn't succeeded, someone asked him, "Are you going to have ten thousand failures?" His response was, "I haven't failed. I've simply discovered 9,999 ways not to invent the electric light bulb."

Most people who achieve anything great have done so by learning from things that do not work. No matter how many times you have been disappointed with other programs, you now have a great opportunity to finally achieve your health and appearance goals by using the Body Contouring Program. Now you've found the way to be successful.

CHAPTER TEN

Postpartum Marriage Conflict

a s Marcia began to tell her story, everyone in this group of women (a Bye-Bye Babyfat support group meeting) could relate. "Everything he did bothered me," she explained, referring to her husband. "He wouldn't help the way he should, and he refused to give me the support and encouragement that I needed."

Marcia's new baby was only three weeks old, and she had a toddler as well. "I was fed up, and I packed all my bags and got the kids and was walking out to the car," she said. "I was leaving him for good. I couldn't stand him. I had loved him before, even a couple of days before, but now he made me ill. He followed me out to the car and tried to grab the baby. We stood there in the driveway, and literally had a tug-of-war with the baby."

Marcia explained that while she could laugh now as she reflected back on this story, it was very serious and upsetting to her at the time. When she finished telling her story (she ended up staying with her husband), almost everyone in the group of twenty women could recall a similar experience one or more times in the first two years after childbirth.

Another group participant, Laura, explained that one week she and her husband felt like their marriage was great, and even talked about how great things were, and the next week she was calling a lawyer to discuss divorce. (They ended up staying together, too.)

Nothing can leave a woman feeling more out of control than a big argument with her husband. When the marriage relationship is in turmoil, nothing else feels secure. Even if you have it together in other areas of your life, marital conflict seems to make everything go sour.

"Our arguments seem to take on a life of their own, and they grow to the point that we are fighting about something completely different than what started it in the first place," Jo Ann said in a postpartum consultation. "Before long I don't even remember how they got started or what triggered them. All I know is that at the time, I feel like he's ruining my life—like I can't stand him! But ten minutes before the argument began I felt like I loved him more than anything in the world. And he might tell me what a great wife I am and that he loves me more than anything, but when an argument starts, he says I never do anything right and he only stays with me because of the baby."

The fact is that both men and women have very high stress levels after the birth of a baby, whether its their first, or one of many, and the postpartum period is one of the most vulnerable times for marriages. It is ironic, too, that women and men often spend so much time on making sure they do every possible thing they believe is in the best interest of their babies, but often they put their marriages on the back burner. In reality, the best thing you can do for a baby is to build a positive, lasting relationship between his or her mommy and daddy.

UNDERSTANDING HIS POSTPARTUM FEELINGS

OBVIOUSLY, it helps to understand your husband's postpartum feelings. Believe it or not, he's experienced some major changes too, and he needs time to adjust. Understanding his feelings might help reduce potential marriage conflict. As all of those who are married know, marriage is a challenge in the best of times. And as all of those who have had a baby know, marriage can be a nightmare during the months and even years after childbirth. If postpartum stress affects every other area of your life, certainly it impacts your marriage. In much the same way that your mind and body must make adjustments after each new baby is born, your relationship with your husband must be adjusted, too.

Arguments are common during periods of high stress—like the postpartum period—and in many cases they could be avoided or minimized if men and women better understood how postpartum stress affects the other.

INTIMACY EQUALS SEX

"HE HAD BEEN GONE on a business trip for six days, and I couldn't wait to share my feelings with him and to tell him all about what the baby, now ten weeks old, had been doing," Samantha explained. "While I was talking to him, I kept noticing him looking over at the television and straining to hear the ballgame. I was crushed, and I sat there feeling so lonely. A little while later he said, "Let's go up to the bedroom while the baby is still asleep." I couldn't believe he even had the nerve to ask me to make love when he couldn't even take a few minutes to talk to me. I just told him he could forget about that idea, and I refused to have sex with him for weeks."

Many of us have probably been surprised by our husband's desire to make love even when we have felt the emotional intimacy was not there. There are good reasons why this type of conflict is so common. Men and women often see things differently. For some men, expressing intimacy means having sex. In other words, the way they feel most comfortable expressing their feelings of love is through sexual closeness. A man might think he's showing his wife that he wants to be close to her by suggesting they make love.

But a woman doesn't see it that way. She desires emotional intimacy, affection, and deep conversation, in order to feel like being physically close. She believes that having sex without emotional closeness is not a true expression of love, but selfish gratification.

According to Dr. Willard F. Harley, Jr., a licensed clinical psychologist, marriage counselor, and author of *His Needs, Her Needs: Building an Affair-Proof Marriage,*[9] the number-one need

---

[9]Willard F. Harley, Jr. *His Needs, Her Needs: Building an Affair-Proof Marriage.* (Tarrytown, New York: The Fleming H. Revell Company, 1986)

of a husband is sexual fulfillment. This need is not necessarily a selfish desire for personal sexual gratification, but a need to bring pleasure to his wife in a way that only he can, and in a way in which he feels comfortable. He needs physical closeness before he feels emotionally connected. Many couples abstain from sexual relations during the final weeks of pregnancy and for six weeks or more after the baby is born. Often, the new mother is so fatigued and consumed with her baby that sex is the last thing on her mind for months after delivery. She might even make the mistake of letting her husband know that sex is the last thing on her mind.

If this sexual "dry spell" goes on very long, her husband might grow very distant emotionally. He might interpret her lack of interest in sex as rejection, and withdraw from his wife. Without sexual relations, he really doesn't know how to be close to his wife. From his point of view, he desires sexual relations because he loves his wife. He probably doesn't understand that women think differently. If she has no interest in sex, he thinks she has no interest in him, and must not really love him.

From the woman's point of view, things are quite different. Many women crave emotional intimacy with their husbands—during the postpartum period more than ever. She wants to feel close to him emotionally, and for her that means having intimate conversations, and sharing thoughts and feelings. She needs this type of closeness in order to feel secure with her new family—to feel like her husband really loves her and is committed. She expresses her love for him by confiding in him, and by telling him her deepest feelings. If he fails to relate to her in this way, she might interpret this as lack of love. If the emotional aspect is present, then the environment is created that makes her feel like making love.

But he desires the sexual environment to draw him out emotionally. Ideally, these two would work together. He showers her with emotional intimacy, listens to her feelings and shares his own, then she feels so close to him that she desires him physically, and feels like making love. But according to

Dr. Harley, a successful marriage counselor who has helped hundreds of couples for more than twenty years, "The typical wife doesn't understand her husband's deep need for sex any more than the typical husband understands his wife's deep need for affection. Affection is the environment of the marriage, and sex is the special event."

In reality, the husband often fails to engage in emotional intimacy, so his wife does not feel like making love, and both go away with their needs unmet. If this withholding continues, resentment and bitterness develop between husband and wife. The pent-up tension and pain they feel often manifests itself in arguments which rage out of control—or result in neglect.

One of the partners in the marriage, either the wife or the husband, must take action to prevent this withholding cycle from taking over. All it takes is to be the one to voluntarily meet the other person's need first. If you start to understand his need to be sexually close, you can begin to express interest in him sexually even if it's the last thing on your mind. Actions precede feelings. In other words, if you express physical desire for him even though you don't feel like it at the time, the feelings will probably come as a result of your taking action.

That doesn't mean you have to have sexual intercourse. We certainly don't recommend having intercourse before your doctor says it's okay. Most husbands understand that you can't have sexual intercourse until you're completely healed. But even during the first six weeks after delivery, you can find ways to let him know that you still find him sexually attractive, and that you are looking forward to resuming that part of your relationship. You can snuggle with him and make him feel like you really want him. This is one of the few special parts of your life with your husband that the new baby can't take over.

Most husbands crave physical closeness with their wives as soon as is reasonable after childbirth, because they've missed the

> *Most husbands understand that you can't have sexual intercourse until you're completely healed. But even during the first six weeks after delivery, you can find ways to let him know that you still find him sexually attractive.*

physical closeness and need reassurance that this aspect of the relationship is still important to you. Husbands often feel jealous of the focus and attention you give the new baby. They feel they've taken a back seat, and it is up to us to find ways to let them know they're still important.

ATTENTION EQUALS LOVE

RECENTLY, I had a very interesting experience with a man I didn't even know. One of my postpartum clients, who had been to the clinic to see me several times, called me and asked if I could do her a favor. She wanted to know if I would consider meeting with her husband. She said that I had helped her a great deal with her postpartum stress, but that he wasn't handling the experience too well, and that was causing problems between the two of them.

It was becoming more and more clear to me that we needed to address male/female relationship conflict in this postpartum book, and so I decided to meet with him at my office. Although I had met with other husbands, I wasn't sure how much I could help him, but I was certain I could learn from him. So he made an appointment and came to see me. As we sat there and talked, I became more and more intrigued with him. Nothing about the way he related his problems to me was anything like the way his wife had explained them. Jim had very little interest in discussing conflict in his marriage or anything of a personal nature. He had withdrawn. Apologetically, he explained to me that his work was the most important part of his life.

"She's got the baby to keep her busy, and I'm just focused on my business—it's number one for me. I know that's not the way it's supposed to be, but that's the way it is," Jim explained.

As we continued to talk, Jim's real feelings began to surface. It turned out that since the baby was born, he felt like his wife had stopped paying attention to him, and he was hurt. At work, he was the boss and got a lot of attention and admiration.

So he had shifted his focus to the place where he felt wanted—to the place where he could get his needs met. I think Jim's response is typical for many men. Rather than express their hurt feelings to their wives, men will often suppress them and simply turn their focus away from home and toward work or something or someone else. Unfortunately, many of us as mothers forget to pay special attention to our husbands after our babies are born.

When husbands are accustomed to being the focus of their wives' attention, and they suddenly have to take a back seat to the baby, they might feel like we don't love them anymore. After all, when you first fell in love with your husband, how did you express that love? Probably, you noticed every little thing he did. You paid attention to what he said, what he did, what he had on—everything. You probably loved just sitting next to him, touching him, and being close. You praised him and were impressed by him. All these things told him you loved him—and he felt fulfilled. If we stop doing most of these things after a baby is born, he might interpret the lack of attention as lack of love.

It is very important to remind ourselves that our marriage—our relationship with our husbands—is the primary relationship. The greatest gift we can give our children is a sound relationship between "mommy and daddy." The children are a manifestation of each partner's love for the other. Both your baby and your husband crave your love and attention. Your baby will let you know if she's not getting enough—your husband might not. But you can meet his need for your attention by taking a little time each day to focus on him. Get a babysitter and let him know you want to go out alone with him on the weekends.

Try to be sensitive to his needs and you will notice when he feels left out. Take time to play with him, and to participate in activities that he enjoys. Look at him the way you did when you first fell in love—and respond to him with loving appreciation for who he is and what he does.

11

C H A P T E R   E L E V E N

For Men Only— How Daddy Can Help!

By Dr. Michael Trexler

I'm leaving you Bill," Ellen shouted as she headed out the front door. "You never talk to me and you just don't care about my feelings. You're an arrogant, self-centered jerk, and I've had it with you!" she added as she slammed the front door.

"What are you talking about?" Bill yelled, as he threw open the door and followed her out to the car. She put the baby in her car seat and got in the car. Bill held the car door open and continued to rage. "I bend over backwards for you, but nothing's good enough," he complained. "I'm glad you're leaving. You're crazy. Superman couldn't please you."

Just thirty minutes earlier, Bill had commented to Ellen how great it was to have their new baby and to be a real family. It had been five weeks since their baby girl was born, and from Bill's perspective, things couldn't be better. He was actually feeling proud of himself. He thought he had really been helping out, and he was enjoying his new role as daddy.

But there was something Bill didn't understand at the time. Ellen was feeling neglected. From her perspective, Bill had been unwilling to meet her needs at all. She had tried several times during the past few days to sit down and tell him how she was feeling, and each time he had tuned her out and remained focused on the television set. This particular day, she tried once again to talk to him—to no avail. She couldn't take it anymore. This man that she needed so desperately to communicate with and be close to seemed as cold as a stone. Yet, he had no clue she wanted to say anything to him that couldn't wait until "nothing good" was on TV. Hurt and anger had been building up inside Ellen for weeks. She couldn't believe she was married to such an insensitive man. How could there be such a discrepancy in the way this couple perceived their situation? The answer is that most men and women have completely different ideas about what it means to be helpful. Since their daughter was born, Bill had picked up some groceries when Ellen asked him to, and he had even thrown an occasional load of laundry into the washing machine. He had made his own lunches (Ellen used to make his lunch), and remembered to take out the garbage. Bill was positive that he was pitching in above and beyond the call of duty, and in fact, he was doing some helpful things.

But he didn't realize that he was completely overlooking Ellen's most desperate postpartum needs—her need for his attention and affection, and her need to have deep conversations with him. He didn't even realize that he was ignoring her when she would try to talk to him about her day, or share with him something about how she was feeling. He wasn't intentionally trying to hurt her, yet to her it felt like he had withdrawn emotionally when she needed him most. She felt lonely and isolated, and she needed Bill's attention. Ellen needed to be emotionally close to him. Sure, helping out around the house was important, but to Ellen it was not nearly as important as getting the emotional intimacy she craved.

Bill is not a bad guy. He had a genuine desire to be helpful. He just didn't know how to help his wife in ways that met her needs. He thought since he was doing a few extra things, he was really helping. If he had known what Ellen needed, he could have responded to her more effectively. The fact is, based on our experience working with postpartum women, the majority of men do not understand their wives' special emotional needs during the weeks and months after childbirth.

All too often, a woman has difficulty expressing these needs to her husband in a way that he can understand. Instead, she might become critical and resentful toward him because she feels neglected. Instead of sitting down and explaining her feelings and what she needs from him (often, she doesn't even understand at the time) she picks on him for every little thing, or explodes at him in anger. This makes him withdraw even more—and the results can be very destructive.

Hey guys, I'll be the first to admit that I was taken by surprise when my method of trying to "help" Sandy resulted in criticism and tears on her part. Finally, I had to learn what my wife wanted and needed from me, and then I had to learn how to give it to her. It was tough! I had always been used to doing things my way. I had the "do your own thing" mentality. But this selfish type of thinking was hurtful to Sandy, and consequently, it was detrimental to me. When I learned to give her more of what she needed—attention, affection, and conversation—I found that I almost always received significant returns on my investment! She would bend over backward to try and please me, instead of criticizing or picking on me. A little understanding about what she needed helped me create a win/win situation in our home. If someone as insensitive as I was could improve, you can do it, too.

In the following pages I have outlined what I've learned, through personal experience as well as the experiences of our clients, about the special needs women have after childbirth. I'm not a marriage counselor or a therapist, but I am a husband and a father who cares about his family. As a health professional, I know that turmoil in your marriage can be very damaging to your mental and physical health. It can cause significant setbacks in your wife's postpartum recovery as well—and that affects the entire family. I believe that the understanding I've gained about women's postpartum needs will help other men meet the needs of their wives during this special time. In an attempt to share this information, we will explore two distinct areas and answer the questions that most men have:

> *When I learned to give her more of what she needed—attention, affection, and conversation—I found that I almost always received significant returns on my investment!*

1 What's happening to my wife during the postpartum period, and what is she feeling?

2 What are her needs, and how can I meet them?

WHAT'S HAPPENING TO MY WIFE, AND WHAT IS SHE FEELING?

1 She is physically and emotionally exhausted.

Wouldn't you be? Think about it for a minute. She just went through nine months of pregnancy and might have gained thirty, forty, or more pounds. In addition to the process of growing a new life inside her body for nine months, she went through some intense pain and physical trauma during labor and delivery. Did you watch?

Our wives deserve a gold medal for enduring that kind of ordeal. If that's not enough, immediately after giving birth, a new mom has constant responsibility for the care of this new baby. And that's a twenty-four-hour-a-day job! Her fatigue is magnified due to a lack of sleep—because she is probably getting up to feed the baby several times a night.

> *O*ur wives deserve a gold medal for enduring that kind of ordeal. If that's not enough, immediately after giving birth, a new mom has constant responsibility for the care of this new baby.

Her emotions also are at a peak. Many men might not understand that their wives often feel a sense of loss after the baby is born. The life that she carried inside her body is not there anymore. She and the baby have changed from being one, to becoming two separate people. This separation is difficult for some women. Hormones are also readjusting and emotions are affected by these changes. All these changes are natural adjustments that your wife must endure. Since she is physically and emotionally drained, she needs you to be strong, supportive, involved, and protective.

2 Her self-image and body image are different.

Just after childbirth, the way a woman views herself and her body changes. Often, the changes are temporary, but nonetheless real at the time. After the draining experience of childbirth, the typical woman does not feel very attractive. She is in pain, her breasts are engorged and leaky, and she is carrying around extra weight.

Her role changes as well, as she becomes consumed with caring for a newborn. If this is her first baby, there is a tremendous change as she adjusts to becoming a mother. And all of us "poor" husbands think we have problems. Our wives have probably gone through much more with pregnancy and childbirth than we ever will. When men accept this fact, we can become truly empathetic and responsive to our wives' postpartum needs.

3 She feels more stress.

Of course this is a general statement, but while both husband and wife experience extra stress with the birth of a new baby, she feels more! Her life changes more than her husband's, and she is the one who must recover physically. When stress levels increase for any family member (or for all family members), conflict becomes more likely. Arguments might quickly rage out of proportion during stressful times. Avoiding damaging arguments is the responsibility of the husband during the weeks and months after your baby is born. Why? Because it might take six months or longer for your wife's physical and emotional changes caused by pregnancy and childbirth to get back to normal.

By giving your wife grace during this time, you will provide a stable, positive influence on your family. Nobody's perfect, but if your goal is to have a peaceful, loving home environment, it takes extra effort on your part. It's much more difficult to be strong, admit your mistakes, say you're sorry, and do what it takes to resolve the conflict. The easy way out is to get mad, argue, and/or walk away. Don't cop out when the going gets tough. The more difficult course of action almost always holds the greatest reward!

I once heard a very unhappy, 240-pound ex-football player say, "I won the argument, but I lost my wife and family." There are no winners in "uncontrolled, anything goes" types of arguments. There's always damage left to be repaired. Sometimes, the damage is too great to repair easily. Small dings in the side of your car door can be easily repaired, but if you have a head-on collision, the damage might be irreparable. Slow down, think, and eliminate the head-on collisions in your marriage.

4 She feels isolated and needs attention.

After a woman delivers her baby, all the attention from others, including the husband, shifts away from her and to the new baby. At first, this attention shift might not be noticed by the mother because she, too, is caught up in the excitement surrounding the baby. However, after a few days, the new mom might feel isolated and neglected.

There are several reasons why she might feel this way. She is no longer the focal point of the "baby" experience. Just before the baby was born, the very pregnant mom was seeing her doctor every week. She was encouraged during these visits, and everyone seemed interested in her progress. Her husband, friends, and relatives were all focused on her—on how she was doing and how she felt. After delivery, everyone's focus shifted from mom to baby.

One of our clients, Tammy, said, "Steve was so complimentary of my appearance during the last weeks of my pregnancy. He said I had a radiant glow and was more beautiful than ever. But after our baby was born, I never heard a single compliment about me. I needed his approval and attention then more than ever—because I felt ugly. I needed to hear him say that he still found me attractive."

Steve missed a golden opportunity to make his wife feel more attractive and more secure! Husbands often fail to sincerely compliment their wives during normal times. It's even more important to recognize her need in this area during the postpartum period.

5 Our Wives Gave It All!

After delivery, a woman is painfully aware that she has just given her all for her husband. She sacrificed her body for nine months during pregnancy and for several more months after delivery so that the two of you could have a family. She had to give totally of herself. Physically, she gained extra weight, monitored everything she ate, endured great pain, and did many other things that help develop a healthy baby. If we as husbands don't acknowledge these sacrifices, she feels taken for granted. She might not say anything about it, but the hurt is there. Our wives need us to appreciate the sacrifices they make in providing us with a new and special miracle.

To quickly review some common feelings reported by wives after childbirth, let's look at the following list.

- She is physically and emotionally exhausted.

- She feels less attractive, and her self-image and body image has changed.

- She feels stressed.

- She feels isolated.

- She gave it all!

If these are the feelings she is likely experiencing, what does she need from her husband? Read on!

WHAT ARE HER NEEDS AND HOW CAN I MEET THEM?

HUSBANDS MIGHT FORGET that it is their responsibility to find out what their wives need and then meet those needs. Ideally, under normal circumstances, it works both ways. If two people are truly committed to each other, and desire a fulfilling and lasting relationship, then they both work to meet each other's needs.

However, during the postpartum period, your wife's needs are the top priorities. She has been sacrificing for nine months and is now faced with the challenge of meeting all the needs of a totally dependent infant. Her resources for meeting your needs might be exhausted for a while, and she needs you to help her regain her physical and emotional strength and energy. Everyone has a certain amount of emotional energy stored up inside. If your reserves are depleted, it becomes difficult to give anymore. Pregnancy, delivery, and all the responsibilities of being a new mom have depleted her reserves, and she needs you to help her build them back up. Remember, pregnancy and delivery were her times to sacrifice. During the postpartum period, it's your turn.

Husbands might forget that it is their responsibility to find out what their wives need and then meet those needs.

One of the ways you can help your wife recover is to be understanding and avoid upsetting or angering her during this stressful time. The most commonly reported things men do (or don't do) that create hurt feelings in their wives during the postpartum period are listed as follows:

- Men don't engage in conversation.

- Men don't actively listen to their wives (by giving eye contact, turning off the TV, etc.)

- Men act uncaring or apathetic regarding their wives' feelings or needs.

- Men are defensive or have a tendency to blow up at any hint of criticism.

- Men don't demonstrate enough affection (through special attention or compliments).

I realize that although men are not perfect, most have good intentions. Most men would like to be more sensitive to their wife, but it just takes so much effort, and it goes against their natural tendencies. For many men, it doesn't come naturally to want to sit down and have intimate conversations, or to demonstrate affection the way your wife would like for you to do. The result is that you might end up hurting your partner's feelings. It might seem at times like you can't win—that there is no use in trying.

A friend of mine, Rick, once confided to me, "Mike, I'm just going to stop trying to please Jill. She gets mad every time I try to do something nice for her. Last week, I asked her to get a baby sitter because I wanted to take her out and spend time with her. She had been complaining that all I ever wanted to do on the weekends was sit in front of the TV. So she got a sitter, and we went out. Right in the middle of the evening, she just got up and wanted to leave. She was in tears and said she was having a terrible time. I couldn't believe it. Nothing could please her."

As we continued our discussion, Rick explained that he had taken her to a basketball game. I cringed because I had made the same mistake about three years earlier. I took Sandy to a Dallas Mavericks game for her birthday. The irony of this was that we had been arguing for the previous few weeks because she felt I watched too much basketball. However, the way I saw it, this would be different because we would go to a game together instead of my watching basketball on TV. So I couldn't understand why, in tears, she wanted to get up and leave at half time. (I thought maybe it was because the Mavericks were playing so poorly. I almost cried myself!)

I later found out she was looking forward to a romantic dinner and a night of intimate conversation to celebrate her birthday. Attending a basketball game was not her idea of the ideal birthday evening. I can look back now and see how thoughtless it was. But at the time, I really thought she would be as excited about going to that basketball game as I was. Almost everyone has a tendency to relate to others or do for others based on what we value, or what would please us. But Rick and I both learned a valuable lesson—if you want to please your wife, get to know what she likes. Her idea of a great night out is probably quite different from yours.

■ WHAT SHE NEEDS FROM YOU

IF YOU LOOK BACK at the list of things men do to create hurt feelings, you will notice a common theme: Men don't communicate very well. Many of us are plagued with a macho attitude that encourages us to be cool and unresponsive. I have been as guilty as anyone, and I'm really trying to improve. Not communicating well or not putting out the necessary effort to respond to your partner is, for the most part, selfish.

The hardest thing for me to do was to look honestly at my behavior and admit to myself and to Sandy that I was weak in my skills of communication with her, although communication from a business perspective is one of my greatest skills—it's what I do for a living. When I admitted my weaknesses on this personal level, she responded very positively. She loved the fact that I was concerned enough about our relationship to look closely at my own behavior. She also was happy that I was taking responsibility by admitting my faults to her. By just making this simple effort, our relationship improved.

I was amazed. I didn't have to make more money, or take out the trash, or do the dishes. I just talked openly and honestly with her. Here's my point: Doing things, or performing for your wife is less important than being emotionally in touch with her on a daily basis. Now, if you spice up your communication by giving her sincere and frequent compliments, and by paying special attention to her, you will most likely spark a tremendous boomerang effect. You will get back much more than you invested. It's like compounding interest at 50 percent. If you could get that kind of return in business, you would likely invest everything you've got.

Well, in your personal life, this high return is almost guaranteed, if you make the investment. So what does your wife need from you and how can you meet those needs? Here are some commonly reported postpartum needs and ways you can respond.

HER NEED: She needs to hear how great she did during pregnancy, labor, and delivery. Think about how you would feel if you won an Olympic gold medal in your favorite sport. You would expect some acknowledgment and praise. She has successfully completed an even greater event. She's been through training, completed the event, and now she needs to be rewarded. She needs your praise.

YOUR RESPONSE: Praise your wife. Tell her in many different ways how great she did and that you are proud of her. Tell her you don't see how she did it, and let her know you are impressed. Admire her for this accomplishment, and tell her what you're thinking.

HER NEED: She needs to know that she's still number one in your life and that you think she's more attractive and desirable than ever.

YOUR RESPONSE: Tell her she's the most important thing in your life, and that nothing else even compares. Let her know that in your eyes, she is the most beautiful woman on earth, and compliment her specifically. Does she have beautiful eyes? Tell her. Maybe you love her smile or something else. Let her know. Make her feel that you desire her even if it's too soon to make love. All these things will help rebuild her self-esteem.

HER NEED: She needs you to show her affection and attention and show her you really care for her.

YOUR RESPONSE: Kiss her when you wake up in the morning and several times during the day. Leave her a little note several times a week, just to say you're thinking about her or that she's doing a great job and you love her. Give her an unexpected hug every chance you get. Phone her from work just to see how she's doing, and tell her you miss her. Bring her a flower, or send her flowers from work. Tell her you love her every day. All these things build the security she craves after childbirth.

HER NEED: She needs you to be interested in what she says. She needs you to listen closely (eye contact and full attention) when she's speaking to you, and to be alert and responsive.

YOUR RESPONSE: Act enthusiastic or at least interested when she tells you anything. Stop what you're doing, put down the newspaper, and become involved in the conversation. Ask probing questions, such as "What did you do today?" "How are you feeling?" or "What could I do to make things easier on you?" Ask follow-up questions based upon her responses.

HER NEED: She needs you to share your feelings with her.

YOUR RESPONSE: Tell her you'd like to sit down and talk. Share some of the feelings you have about her, about the baby, or others. Tell her how much you love your new family, etc. Don't talk about sports, the house, or the weather. Talk about things that are special between you and her.

HER NEED: She needs praise and encouragement for little things as well as major things.

YOUR RESPONSE: Comment on little things she's done that day, or things she is doing. Tell her the coffee is extra good today, or the dinner she prepared was excellent. Notice if she's fixed her hair or had time to put on real clothes. Notice how well she handles being a mom and a wife. If she is working, compliment her on how well she manages all her responsibilities.

HER NEED: She needs to be able to tell you her feelings no matter what they are. If she's irritable, she needs for you to be understanding. You might feel like she's picking on you, but there is probably something deeper that is bothering her. Find out what it is, and provide support. She needs to have confidence in you, that you won't get mad and defensive.

YOUR RESPONSE: Encourage her to tell you how she feels about anything—even if she is upset with you. Remain calm and interested. Ask her to tell you more about how she feels, and then ask specifically what she needs for you to do. If she says she needs you to do something, do it. Remember, this is investment time. Long-term rewards await you.

HER NEED: She needs you to notice when she's down.

YOUR RESPONSE: Encourage her to get her feelings out. Observe her and notice if her mood changes or if she becomes withdrawn. Ask her if there is something bothering her, and if she would share it with you. Don't get frustrated. She needs you to stay with it and draw her out until she feels better. Never, never, never walk out on her or even away from her when she's hurting. She interprets this as abandonment, and in the context of what she's been through, she can't handle that type of behavior. If she retreats to the bedroom, follow her. Help her get through this confusing time. You're the only one who can!

HER NEED: She needs you to think she's doing a great job with the baby.

YOUR RESPONSE: Tell her she's the world's greatest mom. Compliment her on how well the baby is doing. Give her the credit. She has earned it.

HER NEED: She needs to know that you are a shield of protection and security for her and the baby.

YOUR RESPONSE: Act responsibly. Don't spend your free time away from home. She needs you at home. Use your free time to give her breaks. Tell her and show her that you will take care of her and the baby.

HER NEED: She needs your support as she begins the Body Contouring Program found in this book.

YOUR RESPONSE: Tell her you are proud of her for her commitment to improving her health through the Body Contouring Program. Help her find time to complete the exercises each day.

This message is aimed specifically at husbands: You are the single greatest influence on your wife's overall happiness during the postpartum period.

Some men blame hormones, lack of sleep, job pressures, or even their other children for their wives' unhappiness. I would bet that these husbands are not actively attempting to understand and meet their wives' needs. What a great honor, when you really think about it, that your wife places so much importance on your relationship. It is actually a good feeling to be needed in this way.

I've heard many men say, "Hey, I'm tired, too; I can't do it all myself." That might be true. But I don't care what you are doing, you are not as tired as she is, and it actually takes very little effort for you to do the things we've mentioned which help her most. You can do it. She needs time to recover, and she needs your help. Don't forget, you had a big role in creating this event—so see it through. Daddies can be a big help!

To close out this man-to-man talk, I want to share with you some critical steps helpful in stopping arguments before they get out of hand. It's easy to put out the flame of a match, before much damage is done. But if the flame is left burning, it will grow into a raging inferno and even if it is extinguished, the damage is enormous. The same is true with arguments. Extinguish them before they have time to grow.

Most arguments start out quietly and slowly, and are usually based upon some lack of communication or lack of understanding. Usually neither of the two involved ever intended for things to get out of hand. During the progression of these arguments, many extremely hurtful things are often said. Once these things are said, they are difficult to take back; they are damages much like the ones left behind from a raging fire. After these types of damages have been inflicted, things must be rebuilt. Your relationship must be rebuilt each time you have an out-of-control argument—because the damages are severe. Next time you find yourself in the early stages of an argument, don't fan the flame—extinguish it.

Here's how:

- You make the first move as peacemaker. Say, "Let's stop. I don't want to argue with you. I love you. Would you help me understand how you're feeling?"

- You take responsibility for the argument—even if you think it was her fault. Ask yourself if it is more important to be happy or to be right. Most of us would rather be happy, and she will recognize what you did.

- Apologize and tell her you love her and your goal is to understand her better. "I'm sorry" almost always works!

- Don't jump back into the argument. Refuse to say another destructive word.

- Do not walk away. Stick with her until the conflict is resolved.

There is a universal principle that goes like this: When you're willing to act unselfishly and express concern for the needs of another out of love, you always get back much more than you gave. I honestly believe you get back ten times more. In other words, if you focus on your wife's needs at the expense of your own, you will find your needs met in ways you never imagined. It might not happen immediately, but you will reap the rewards in the long run. You can't give too much to your wife during the postpartum period.

Body Contouring Principles

Dr. Michael Trexler

PART TWO

II

CHAPTER TWELVE

Postpartum Perfect

*N*ew mothers: It's never too late to start reshaping your body and losing that excess babyfat after pregnancy. Nor is it ever too early to start. In fact, we recommend that you begin this Body Contouring Program as soon as possible after delivery.

This is a program that combines healthy, low-fat eating with the proper type of low-intensity exercise to achieve permanent fat loss and toned, shapely muscles. This is not too good to be true. What you accomplish is all up to you. The thing to keep in mind is body contouring. We call it body contouring because even if you are only five pounds overweight, your body's contour, shape, and appearance is adversely affected.

Five pounds of excess fat can alter the size of your waist— so much so that your clothes are uncomfortably tight. It can latch on to the outside of hips and thighs, thus giving you a wider appearance, and it can produce a dimpling effect commonly called cellulite (which is really just stored fat, and can only be eliminated by losing the fat).

Fat sits on top of your muscles. That's why even if you have shapely, toned muscles underneath the fat, they don't show. If five pounds of excess fat tissue stored in your body can affect its shape and appearance, think about what fifteen pounds, twenty-five pounds, or more can do! It conceals your natural, beautiful body contour. It's time for you to lose this stubborn fat tissue, and reveal your healthy shape. We say healthy shape because losing this fat not only enhances your appearance, it improves your health even more! It is natural to gain some fat during pregnancy. But it's not natural, and it's very unhealthy, to continue to carry it around for the rest of your life.

This program is the safest, most effective way to lose your pregnancy-related babyfat!

Just before our baby, Michael, was born, Sandy was looking forward to giving birth and getting her figure back. She had gained about forty pounds during pregnancy, although she exercised and ate a high-quality, low-fat diet. We were both surprised at how much weight she gained.

Just a few days before her delivery, I tried to reassure Sandy by saying, "It will all be over soon and all that weight will be gone; I'm sure you'll feel much better then!" I really believed that most of Sandy's extra weight would disappear shortly after birth—and I had convinced her, too. After all, she had done all the right things throughout her pregnancy: regular exercise, good diet, no alcohol, no caffeine, not even prescription drugs. As a matter of fact, she did all the right things even before she was pregnant. So I thought this extra weight was all related to the baby.

Sandy focused on how great it would feel to fit into her size-five jeans again. (Of course, our main focus was always on having a healthy baby. We both prayed daily that Sandy's delivery would go well and that our baby would be perfect. As it turned out, we were blessed!)

But as her due date got closer, Sandy began to be concerned that her weight gain might not disappear immediately after delivery. She had been reading in her pregnancy books that only twelve to fifteen pounds would be lost with delivery of the baby and maybe another five pounds over the next few days. A little quick math and we estimated that she would be left with an "extra" twenty pounds. But I had it figured out. Our baby would be a strapping twenty-pounder! To support such a big guy the placenta would be about ten pounds and the fluid loss with delivery would be seven pounds. I said, "Sweetheart, you really only gained three pounds!"

I then explained my twenty-pound-baby theory to her. Needless to say, she was not overjoyed with the thought of giving birth to a twenty-pound baby. (Note to husbands: Do not use the word "baby" and twenty pounds in the same sentence!) A few days later, Michael was born—eight pounds, six ounces. Our doctor said that was the largest baby Sandy could have delivered vaginally. She had required a fourth-degree episiotomy, which is the most severe. However, she felt pretty good with a new little boy in her arms. We both were so happy.

I still don't know why, but there was a weight scale just down the hall. The scale just seemed so menacing. What could the hospital people be thinking? Was this their idea of a cruel joke? Then I got off the scale. I guess I was a little frustrated with my own fifteen-pound "sympathy" weight gain. After all, I wasn't the one pregnant.

Sandy was on the scales the next day. "I can't believe it," she exclaimed. "I'm still twenty pounds overweight, and I look six months pregnant!" Never at a loss for words, I stammered, "Uh, well, Honey, duh—no you don't, you look great." She did look beautiful to me, but it was obvious that her current physical condition was a major concern to her.

Sandy wanted to find a role model who had been through pregnancy and childbirth and who had been successful at getting her figure back. Although many general exercise and weight-loss books were available, we couldn't find one that offered a comprehensive postpartum program which considered the unique needs a woman has after childbirth. After all, many things are different for the mom during this time.

Because Sandy and I both have had great success at helping people lose weight, we decided we would develop a safe and effective program aimed specifically at new mothers and with the goal to help them lose the excess babyfat gained with pregnancy.

HOW DOES THE BODY CONTOURING PROGRAM WORK?

BODY CONTOURING is an activity system that will safely help you achieve a firm, shapely figure and more attractive appearance. This program is based on the scientific principles that explain how the body burns fat the most efficient way. This method of burning body fat also is great for improving your health and keeping you healthy.

Our activity program is based on low-intensity exercise that directly stimulates the fat cells to release fat. Once the fat is released from the storage cells into the bloodstream, it can be taken to the muscles and burned. This is the only way you can get rid of fat! You can't melt it away, sweat it out, or massage it out. It has to be burned in your muscles!

> *Our activity program is based on low-intensity exercise that directly stimulates the fat cells to release fat. Once the fat is released from the storage cells into the bloodstream, it can be taken to the muscles and burned.*

Over the past few years, we've gotten accustomed to aerobics instructors telling us to push a little harder, feel the burn, keep your heart rate in the "target" zone—no pain, no gain. But really, the harder you exercise, the less fat you burn. That's because our muscles use two basic fuels when we exercise: carbohydrates for hard or fast exercise, and fats for slower, easy exercise. Your muscles do not ache or burn when fat is being used for fuel. If you feel the "burn," you are producing lactic acid in the muscles by exercising too hard. Lactic acid is produced by using carbohydrate fuel that's loaded in the muscles. This means that you're not burning fat! You must slow down enough to prevent lactic acid from being produced. *You must go slow to burn fat.* Exercising too hard will prevent fat from being burned.

Our program is highly effective at training your body to release and burn unwanted body fat. Training your body to become efficient at burning fat involves three key factors:

- Exercising at a low to moderate pace for more than twenty minutes, five to six days per week, to turn on your "Fat-Burning Switch"!

- Reducing excess fat in your diet, and eating more carbohydrates. By eating less fat, you will have less to store and less to burn. By eating more carbos, you actually burn fat at a faster rate.

■ Performing light resistance exercise. Very simple, five to ten minutes per day, two to three days per week. This stimulates metabolism and muscle tone. (Carrying around a baby is one form of resistance exercise.)

You probably have seen the advertisements that claim you can get an aerobic workout in as little as twelve minutes a day by using a particular piece of equipment or a certain program. These ads are missing the point. You can improve your fitness level by increasing your muscle strength and heart function, but hardly any fat is burned during these short exercise sessions! If you want to lose fat, thus losing weight, you must exercise at a slower pace for longer periods of time. It sounds great to exercise just twelve minutes three times a week. The truth is, it just doesn't work for fat loss.

Imagine trying to cook your fifteen-pound Thanksgiving turkey in a five-hundred-degree oven in only twelve minutes. Although the oven is hot enough, there just isn't enough heat absorbed by the turkey long enough to fully cook the meat (not even in a microwave). You'll burn up the outside, but the inside will remain raw. Part of the turkey has cooked—but not the right part! However, if you turn down the heat and cook it more slowly for a longer period of time, the meat gets properly cooked—the job gets done the right way and the result is exactly what you desired!

The Body Contouring Program is great for stimulating your body to burn extra fat. It works much like cooking in an oven. Think about what is happening when you preheat an oven. The oven is on and it's working, but it takes time for the oven to get ready to cook. It takes time to reach the proper temperature. You don't begin counting the cooking time until the oven is preheated to the appropriate temperature, then you put the food in, close the door, and start the timer.

Our exercise program allows for your muscles to "preheat" and prepares your fat to be released from its storage tanks. Then your muscles become fat-burning machines. We will teach you how to count and record your Fat Burning Minutes (FBMs). The term Fat Burning Minutes refers to the time you exercise after your body is warmed up or preheated, just as the time you cook something in the oven only begins after the oven is pre-heated to a certain temperature.

Another important point is to enjoy what you're doing. Some people will say, "I just don't enjoy exercising." They are usually referring to the hard, painful type of exercise. But almost everyone enjoys walking, because it is easier and it truly leads to a thinner, more attractive appearance. In our program, you will not only enjoy the exercise, but you'll also enjoy the results!

There are two parts to the Body Contouring Program: Basic and Advanced. Each part is six weeks long. The Basic Program should be completed before beginning the Advanced Program. If you're a working mom, you'll be in good shape when you return to work by completing the Basic Program. (The program's exercise schedules are provided in Appendix 1.)

■ THE BASIC PROGRAM

THE BASIC PROGRAM is the foundation for successful fat loss. Remember, your goal is to lose fat and keep it off for good. For this to happen, you have to (1) train your body to let go of the stored fat, and (2) exercise at the correct pace so your muscles can burn the fat.

■ THE ADVANCED PROGRAM

AFTER COMPLETING THE BASIC BODY CONTOURING PROGRAM, you have two very good options:

■ Option One
Continue your fat-burning activity by following week five or six from the Basic Program. Keep doing the suggested exercises and control fat intake while eating at least fifteen hundred calories per day.

■ **Option Two**

Begin the Advanced Body Contouring Program and achieve higher levels of fitness and enhanced body shape. If you decide to use the Advanced Program, you will speed up the rate of fat loss in your body. It will become easier for your body to burn fat and harder to store fat. The Advanced Program will get you where you always wanted to be and keep you there!

With either option you are dramatically improving your health, appearance, and body shape.

Completing the Basic Program is like completing elementary school, junior high, and high school—all in just six weeks. The Advanced Program is like getting a college degree with honors! The longer you stick with the program, the more dramatic results you'll see!

Some women have asked if they could just start with the Advanced Program so they could get the results faster. Don't do it. It's very unlikely you could get to college without first completing your basic education (elementary, junior high, and high school). It's also unlikely that your fat cells and muscles have been trained properly to allow your body to burn fat effectively. If you complete the Basic Program first, you will benefit much more from the Advanced Program. No train, no gain! By now you might be wondering why it's so hard to burn fat. One reason is because we have so much of it stored in so many places.

FIFTY BILLION FAT STORAGE TANKS ■

MANY PEOPLE DO NOT KNOW that we use different types of fuel for different types of exercise. This fuel comes in three different forms: fat (yes, fat is a fuel), carbohydrates, and protein. It might surprise you, but protein is used very little for fuel or to give you energy. In fact, protein is just a standby or emergency fuel. Protein is mostly used to give the muscles structure or to repair damaged tissue. So, in reality, you only have two sources that supply you with significant amounts of energy—fats and carbohydrates. The fats and carbohydrates that you have available for energy come from the foods you eat.

If you eat a lot of fat, guess what? You get fat! Fat is easily stored inside the body, and the amount stored is almost unlimited. That's because everyone has an incredible number of fat storage tanks. The storage tanks are called fat cells. Each fat cell is an individual storage tank for extra fat.

The average person has between twenty-five billion and seventy-five billion fat cells. Some extremely obese people have well over two hundred billion. This variation in the number of fat cells helps determine your body-shape potential. By late adolescence (age sixteen to seventeen) you basically have all the fat cells you're going to get.

Fat cells do not go away (unless we have them vacuumed out by liposuction—and that's only three to five pounds at about $1000 per pound!). They either shrink or expand as fat is added or drained. Most of your fat cells are located just under the skin (called subcutaneous fat). You know it's there because you can feel it, touch it, and see it! That's the harsh reality. As one of our clients said, "If it would just hide deeper inside my body, that wouldn't be so bad." Maybe not for appearance, but the fact is that having too much fat anywhere in your body is harmful to your health.

Let's say you have an average number of fat cells—fifty billion or so. Picture each of your individual fat cells as balloons. They have the capability of expanding when something is put inside. If you bought a package of one hundred balloons for your baby's first birthday, you could open up the package and hold all those balloons in your hands. Although there are one hundred balloons, they don't take up much space without any air in them.

But what would happen if you blew up all those balloons and then tried to hold them? It would be pretty hopeless; they just take too much space. The balloons now would fill up the entire room! The interesting point is that the number of balloons didn't change—just the size and the amount of space they now take up.

If you eat too much fat and don't exercise correctly to burn it, you will fill up your fat cells in much the same way that air fills up a balloon. The result is that *you* also expand too much and take up more space. Your goal is to help your fat cells release fat so they can shrink and occupy less space.

If you eat too much fat and don't exercise correctly to burn it, you will fill up your fat cells in much the same way that air fills up a balloon.

Almost all of the excess calories you eat beyond what you use daily are converted to fat and stored in your fat cells. Your body needs a certain number of calories every day in order to keep you alive and provide energy for you to move. If you are a breast-feeding mom, you need more calories than you normally would. If you move around a lot, or exercise, you burn more calories, so fewer are left over to be stored as fat. In fact, if you eat fewer calories in a day than you need, then your body borrows some fuel (fat) from your fat storage cells and uses that to keep you going.

This sounds great—just eat fewer calories and you lose weight. Right? Well, not exactly. Several factors are necessary for losing "extra" fat weight: 1) the type of food you eat; 2) the amount of food you eat; and 3) the type of exercise you do. Next, we will explain how you can tap into your fat-burning system. We have to help our fat cells "let go" of the fat and help our muscles burn this "extra" fat that has just been released. To do this, we flip on the "Fat-Burning Switch"!

CHAPTER THIRTEEN

The Twenty-Minute, Fat-Burning Switch: Fat-Burning Minutes

To burn more fat, all you have to do is flip a switch. But first, the flipping-on part requires a little knowledge and a little patience. With help from the Body Contouring Program, you can teach your body how to flip on the switch, preheat your muscles, and burn the excess fat. For your body to use fat for fuel, it must be taken to your muscles and burned. When the fat is burned, guess what? It goes away, and it's gone! This is one of the principles involved in your pledge to say bye-bye to babyfat.

Burning fat is really a simple process. First, you must exercise at the correct speed to nudge your fat cells to release the fat stored inside. Second, you must exercise long enough for the fat to be burned.

Here's how to flip on the Fat-Burning Switch. Walk at a slow, comfortable pace for twenty minutes. At about the twenty-minute mark, the switch is flipped. You switch from burning mostly carbohydrate to fat, and that's what you're after. Every minute beyond twenty minutes burns more and more fat.

The good news is that when you flip on the Twenty-Minute, Fat-Burning Switch, the percentage of fat used for energy goes up. This means if you go for a leisurely paced walk, your fat cells can release more and more fat. Many people believe that exercising for twenty minutes, three times a week, is enough to lose weight. The truth is that twenty minutes is just not enough for you to experience fat loss.

Twenty minutes might be enough to improve or maintain the function of your heart, but it's not enough time to burn extra body fat. If it takes twenty minutes for fat to be released, then we want to take advantage of all the exercise minutes past the twenty-minute mark. That's when we all become fat-burning machines—beyond twenty minutes. So we've now identified two critical factors for really burning up extra body fat!

■ Exercise at a slow and easy pace, without stopping for twenty minutes, to warm up or preheat your body.

■ Continue beyond twenty minutes to get an extra fat-burning boost!

In the past few years, we've been asked many times about this fat-burning-switch idea. A typical question is, "I know we're flipping on the switch to burn more fat, but what are we switching from?"

That's a great question. The answer is carbohydrates. Carbohydrates are stored right inside your muscles. These carbohydrates come from the food you eat, and they are stored in your muscles in the form of glycogen, which is similar to sugar. Your body uses carbohydrates for fast or hard exercise such as running, aerobics, and weight lifting. Any time you are exercising hard enough to cause huffing and puffing or very fast breathing, you are not burning fat. This hard-and-fast type of exercise burns carbohydrates from your muscles.

Slow exercise is required to burn fat. But since you are going slower, the fat calories you use are burning at a slower rate. That's another reason to go beyond twenty minutes; not only do you burn a high percentage of fat, but you burn fat calories for a longer period of time. If your goal is to get rid of extra fat and appear slim and trim, this is the best way to go. We also have included some "booster tips" that accelerate fat loss, even more.

If you have recently gone through pregnancy and childbirth, your fat cells are very good at storing fat. Not only that, they also are extra efficient at holding on to it. It's really hard to force your fat cells to let go, to give up some fat to be burned. (They're stubborn, just like men.)

If you gently persuade the cells to release fat by walking slowly, but continuously, for twenty minutes or more, you will have achieved what you wanted and needed! Your fat cells don't want to give up the fat stored inside, so you have to do the right things to overcome the resistance. If you try to force the fat out of the cells by hard or strenuous exercise, it won't budge. Slow, easy and long does it every time. How long is enough?

FAT-BURNING MINUTES (FBMs)

IN THE FALL OF 1987, while completing the first two years of a four-year Ph.D. program at the University of South Carolina, I was the director of the University's Aerobic Instructor Certification Program. During these two years, I was amazed by the number of aerobics instructors who were dissatisfied with their bodies. Some of these instructors were teaching as many as three classes a day, five days a week, and then working out on their own. It's hard to imagine someone exercising that much and not achieving their weight goals.

After surveying dozens of these instructors I discovered two common elements: 1) Most exercised at a high intensity level five to seven days per week; and 2) many were routinely restricting calories—they didn't eat enough!

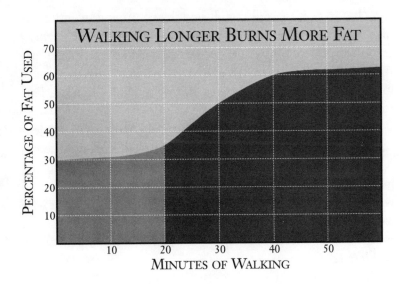

WALKING LONGER BURNS MORE FAT

PERCENTAGE OF FAT USED

MINUTES OF WALKING

It didn't make sense that some were still complaining they were five to ten pounds overweight. I began to understand this mystery as I took a closer look at how the body converts food to fuel. The next step was to learn how our muscles burn the fuel during different types of exercise. After a few months of study, thought, and observation, it became clear. Many people are exercising too hard and not eating enough of the right kinds of food. That's why their bodies hold on to excess fat!

Here's how it works: If you exercise too hard, muscle size usually increases and extra water is sometimes retained. This might add muscle weight and cause a puffy appearance. Also, exercising too hard doesn't directly burn fat calories. When you combine hard or strenuous exercise with a low-calorie (but high-fat) diet, the metabolic boost you should get from the exercise is reduced.

There's simply not enough fuel to keep the muscles hot. Your muscles need to be replenished almost daily with carbohydrates to really boost metabolism. This brings us back to the original point: You have to exercise slower and longer, while eating a higher percentage of carbohydrates and less fat in your diet. It is clear that the longer we exercise at a low-intensity rate the more fat we burn.

It also is fairly well established that at around twenty minutes, the fat-burning rate increases while the rate of burning carbohydrates in the muscle decreases. It makes sense then that the real fat-burning time is after we have been exercising at a low to moderate pace for twenty minutes. Thus, the term, Fat-Burning Minutes (FBMs).

I started using the term Fat-Burning Minutes in my lectures during the spring of 1988. I also advised those instructors who were exercising too hard and too often to reduce the number of their strenuous exercise sessions each week and replace them with walking to get in some FBMs. Those who were eating low-calorie but high-fat diets were advised to eat more carbohydrates (fruits, vegetables, bread, cereal, pasta) and less fat.

Guess what happened? Many reported losing those last few pounds very quickly. Now it made sense. Get in some FBMs and eat a well-balanced diet. Using the information and feedback I had gained, I began to promote walking (rather than running or jogging) as the most efficient way to burn extra body fat. If you can't or don't care to walk, please select one of the other activities we have listed.

In our Body Contouring Program, you gradually, but surely, prepare your fat cells to release fat and your muscles to burn fat. It works great! As you follow our six-week plan, you will gradually accumulate more and more FBMs. We've noticed that most women significantly improve their body shape by working up to 150 FBMs per week. We have outlined a daily schedule to help get you there. (Appendix 1) New moms needn't worry— you start very slowly and you get lots of grace. You deserve it!

IMPORTANCE OF CONTINUOUS WALKING

GAIL, A SUCCESSFUL WEIGHT-LOSS CLIENT, once asked, "What difference does it make if I walk for twenty minutes three times a day, thirty minutes twice a day, or for sixty minutes at one time? After all, I'm getting in the same amount of time, sixty minutes."

For Gail, the main difference was in the total amount of fat burned during those sixty minutes. While the total exercise time was the same, the difference in the number of FBMs was dramatic!

Gail was concerned since she had been walking for twenty minutes three times a day in an attempt to lose weight. First, I applaud anyone who is making that kind of commitment and effort. Gail will get some results if she continues this walking pattern. However, there is a more effective, more direct way to lose body fat. Using Gail's example, let's see how it works.

If you started slowly and gradually increased your pace to a moderate walk, your fat-burning percentage would go up after twenty minutes. After twenty minutes you burn a higher percentage of fat. That's the goal, to burn fat! If you walked for twenty minutes and then stopped, you would just be starting to really burn your excess fat. Remember, at twenty minutes the switch from carbohydrates to fat takes place. Burning fat is like building a campfire; you might spend twenty minutes getting the twigs to heat the sticks to heat the logs long enough until they catch fire.

Let's say it takes twenty minutes to get the logs burning (similar to the twenty minutes it takes to get your fat burning). If you stopped and put the fire out just after you got it burning well, hardly any of the logs would be burned up. (If you stop exercising after only twenty minutes, you put out your fat-burning fire, too!) If you wanted to burn the logs later, you'd have to start the whole process over again. It would take another twenty minutes to get the logs burning. That's why even if you walk three times a day for twenty minutes, you probably won't ever get to your maximum fat-burning percentage. You're putting out your fat-burning fire too early each time.

Although Gail walked for a total of sixty minutes, she didn't get any FBMs. Gail said at first that she just couldn't walk any longer than twenty minutes at a time because she got tired. Gail had been walking too fast over hilly terrain. I advised her to reduce her walking speed and not get out of breath. Look next at the difference in FBMs, if you switch from walking three times a day for twenty minutes to two times a day for thirty minutes. Notice that both methods equal sixty minutes per day.

Another client, Betty, walks two times a day for thirty minutes. As you know, the first twenty minutes of our walking program is designed to flip on the Fat-Burning Switch. Therefore, Betty is only burning fat from the twenty-minute mark to the thirty-minute mark, or a total of ten FBMs. Since she walks twice a day, she has twenty FBMs per day (ten FBM minutes for each of her thirty-minute walks). Now, compared to Gail, Betty has improved her fat-loss efficiency, although walking for the same amount of time as Gail.

MAXIMUM BENEFIT

NANCY WALKS FOR SIXTY MINUTES at one time. The first twenty minutes build the fat-burning fire, just as in Gail's and Betty's walks. But Gail stopped at twenty minutes, and Betty only went for ten more minutes. Nancy continues to walk for forty additional minutes after the twenty-minute mark for a total of forty FBMs!

Results of sixty minutes of walking in our examples:

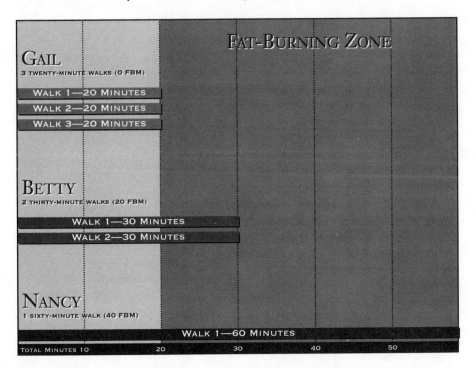

FAT-BURNING ZONE

GAIL
3 TWENTY-MINUTE WALKS (0 FBM)

WALK 1—20 MINUTES
WALK 2—20 MINUTES
WALK 3—20 MINUTES

BETTY
2 THIRTY-MINUTE WALKS (20 FBM)

WALK 1—30 MINUTES
WALK 2—30 MINUTES

NANCY
1 SIXTY-MINUTE WALK (40 FBM)

WALK 1—60 MINUTES

TOTAL MINUTES 10   20   30   40   50

Once you get the fat burning, keep it burning. Go for longer than twenty minutes! The Body Contouring Program is designed to gradually build your strength and endurance so you can walk for longer amounts of time. *Remember, every minute you walk beyond twenty minutes is a Fat-Burning Minute (FBM).*

14

The Body Contouring Program

W elcome to the activity part of our program. In this section we have outlined a day-by-day fat-burning, walking schedule for you to follow. This program works exceptionally well for women who have recently had babies or for those who never lost their weight from previous pregnancies. Our activity program features low-intensity walking. We believe this type of structured walking is the safest and most effective exercise program to use when losing body fat and improving health are the goals.

Before you begin, it's important to ask your medical doctor if there are any reasons why you should not participate in this program. After you obtain your doctor's permission and begin our program, if at any time you experience nausea, dizziness, pain, bleeding, or any other unusual symptom, stop exercising gradually (within one minute) and call your doctor.

Ninety-five percent of women who give birth are advised to get out of bed and walk during the first postpartum day. Even women who had cesareans, episiotomies, or otherwise difficult deliveries are routinely advised to walk. Our Body Contouring Program has been specifically recommended by Ob-Gyn physicians to assist their patients in postpartum recovery.

GETTING STARTED ■

IT'S EASY TO GET STARTED on your "fat reduction" activity program! First, you need a very good pair of walking shoes—not just any shoes, but ones made specifically for exercise walking. These walking shoes are a type of athletic shoes and, like running shoes, are found in sporting goods stores and in some department stores.

Shoe design has improved tremendously in the past few years. Each sport now has shoes that bend and flex with the motions specific to that sport. So, "tennis" shoes are not appropriate for the type of walking that you will be doing. Neither are aerobics shoes, basketball shoes, or even running shoes. At the risk of sounding overbearing, I strongly recommend a pair of athletic walking shoes from your local sporting goods store. Your walking will be more comfortable and, most likely, injury-free if you wear the right shoes!

In addition to walking shoes, you need a good, supportive bra. Ideally, your workout bra will hold your breasts almost stationary while you walk. If you are a C cup or larger, it might be helpful to wear two bras—one on top of the other—during exercise, for extra support. Buy bras specially designed for exercise, or else find regular bras designed to provide "heavy duty" support. Always change into a dry bra immediately after exercise to prevent yeast problems.

USING THE BODY CONTOURING ACTIVITY SCHEDULES

PLEASE COMPLETE THE PRE-CONDITIONING PROGRAM before beginning the Basic Body Contouring Program. The two-week Pre-Conditioning Program can be found in chapter 5. If, however, you are now walking thirty minutes a day at least five days per week, then you can begin with the Basic Program. The schedule guidelines are included in Appendix 1 toward the back of this book. You might wish to place a book marker at Appendix 1, as we'll often refer to the walking schedules in this chapter.

Now the big question: Are you ready to begin? Are you ready to feel better, have more energy, improve your health, and unload all the "extra" babyfat you don't want or need? Okay, here's how to do it! Look at the Week 1 walking schedule in Appendix 1. There are five columns listed:

- Day

- Total Minutes

- Walking Pace

- Fat-Burning Minutes

- Date Completed

Day

THE DAY COLUMN REPRESENTS a seven-day cycle, or a week's worth of activity. You can start on any day of the week; just complete the days in order, one through seven. You can exchange the rest day (Day 5) with Day 4 if you feel like it. Then you would rest on Day 4 and do Day 4's schedule on Day 5.

Total Minutes

THIS COLUMN DISPLAYS the total number of minutes you should walk for the scheduled session. This includes five minutes of slow walking at the beginning and at the end of each session. If you are scheduled to walk for 45 minutes and you begin at 10:00 A.M., you should finish at 10:45 A.M.

Walking Pace

THROUGHOUT THE BODY CONTOURING PROGRAM, you will be asked to walk at varying speeds. This type of paced walking will provide you with the proper stimulation and rest necessary to accelerate fat loss. We measure pace by counting the number of steps you take in fifteen seconds.

From a standstill, take a step with your right foot, that's one. Then take a step with your left foot, that's two. Right foot, three, left foot four, and so on. After many experiments to quantify walking pace, we found that counting the number of steps taken within a certain time was the most practical and effective way to prescribe walking speed and intensity. Here's an easy way to count how many steps you take in fifteen seconds:

- Begin walking without looking at your watch.

■ Practice counting your steps a few times.

■ Start your watch and begin counting your steps.

■ Stop counting when fifteen seconds have elapsed.

If you counted between twenty and twenty-four steps, you were walking at a slow-steady pace. That's our starting pace, good for warming up or slow walking. Here are the paced walking categories:

■ Walking between 20 and 24 steps in 15 seconds is called Slow Pace.

■ Walking between 25 and 29 steps in 15 seconds is called Moderate Pace.

■ Walking between 30 and 34 steps in 15 seconds is called Brisk Pace.

■ And, occasionally, in the Advanced Program, we might ask you to walk at 35 or more steps in 15 seconds. That's called Fast Pace.

Most of the walking in this program is either in the Moderate or Brisk Pace category. You should always begin and end each session with five minutes of Slow Pace.

You will only have to count your steps for a minute or so until you are walking at the proper pace. Then forget about it and enjoy your walk. You might wish to check your walking pace occasionally. Most women find that this type of pacing helps them maintain their motivation throughout the entire walk.

Fat-Burning Minutes (FBMs)

THE NEXT COLUMN REPRESENTS how many Fat-Burning Minutes you get from the total minutes you walk. You can always calculate your FBMs by counting all the minutes you walk past twenty minutes. For example, if you walk for thirty minutes, you get credit for ten Fat-Burning Minutes.

Our goal in the Basic Program is to gradually work up to one hundred fifty FBMs each week. Remember, during the Fat-Burning Minutes, a much higher percentage of body fat is being burned for your exercise fuel! Look at the week-by-week FBMs totals; you get more and more each week. You become a fat-burning machine! (When I lecture on this, if I notice that the "audience" has a good sense of humor, I say, "You become a fat-burning momma!" Sometimes I even get a chuckle out of the serious moms, too!)

Date Completed

THIS COLUMN PROVIDES SPACE to record or check off the date when you complete the schedule for that day. It can provide an incentive or motivation to "just do it," as the Nike ads say. Over the past couple of years I've developed a new motto after hearing the hundreds of reasons, or excuses, why people don't follow through with their exercise programs:

"DO IT ANYWAY!"

Successful people somehow find a way to do it and get the results they're after. Most find success only after trying many, many times. Keep trying and one day it'll happen, and probably a lot sooner than you think! Remember the little train going up the hill, "I think I can, I think I can, I think I can"? Well, say that to yourself, achieve your goal and then say, "I knew I could, I knew I could, I knew I could!"

Before you begin, check these Body Contouring guidelines:

Get your medical doctor's permission.

Wear good quality athletic "walking" shoes.

Drink water before and after your walk.

Don't get out of breath or huff and puff.

Don't get too hot.

If you get dizzy or feel pain, slow down, then stop.

■ Complete the Pre-Conditioning Program before starting the Basic Program.

■ Complete the Basic Program before starting the Advanced Program.

■ You must complete the weekly schedule before you move to the next week. If you miss one day of scheduled walking, repeat the entire week. You're not really getting behind—and you'll get better results in the long run.

■ QUESTIONS AND ANSWERS ABOUT BEGINNING

QUESTION: I can't walk very easily where I live; the traffic is heavy, I don't feel safe, and in the winter it's much too cold. What can I do?

ANSWER: In an ideal world we could just stroll out of our house and down a nice country road in perfect weather. Since things are not always ideal, we need some good options. One option is to get a walking treadmill for your home. Motorized treadmills, are more popular because of huge price reductions in recent years. Many large retail stores (Wal-Mart, Kmart, Sears, JCPenney, and others) offer a variety of good quality treadmills often starting for as low as $200. Expect to pay $700-$800 for top-of-the-line home models.

If you live in a high traffic area, you probably have a large mall or indoor shopping center nearby. Some malls even have walking clubs where members walk together at certain times. Many malls also are smoke-free, making them healthy places to walk as well, and at no charge!

QUESTION: Why is the Body Contouring Program based on walking? Why is walking so good?

ANSWER: Because paced walking will give you the most beneficial results. The reason is that walking tones and shapes muscles in the hip, thigh, and calf areas while stimulating the release of stored fat. Because walking also produces the best possible conditions for the burning of fat, you lose the right type of weight. Also, walking stimulates the production of additional bone density in your legs, hips, and pelvic areas—while reducing stress injuries commonly found in running and high-impact "aerobics." And, as a side effect, your risks of developing high blood pressure, heart disease, and even some forms of cancer are greatly reduced!

QUESTION: I've really tried, but I just can't find a way to walk as often as the program recommends. Is there another exercise I can do to get the same results?

ANSWER: Maybe, but it takes a great deal of commitment, effort, and some experimenting to find an equivalent exercise. One method is to ride a stationary bike at a setting you can maintain for the same number of minutes as prescribed in the Body Contouring walking program. The key is to not get out of breath or cause fatigue or burning in your upper leg muscles.

Another method is outdoor bike riding. However, with outdoor riding there's normally quite a bit of coasting and stopping and starting. So double the number of minutes recommended in the walking schedules to ensure a significant amount of "Fat Burn" when you ride outdoors.

One problem I've observed with bike riding is the uncomfortable feeling of sitting on the seat, especially for women who have recently given birth. Check with your doctor before riding, and wear padded bike shorts on a padded seat, and always wear a helmet. Personally, I'm not in favor of taking your baby along for a ride. It's too dangerous and not worth the risks.

QUESTION: How about aerobics classes or swimming, instead of walking? Aren't these fat-burning exercises?

ANSWER: Not really. Most aerobics instructors urge you to achieve a predetermined target heart rate. Normally, the exercise intensity is too high for fat to be used as the primary fuel source, therefore muscle fuel, or glycogen, is mostly used. Most aerobics classes are designed to improve fitness levels and not necessarily to lose weight. Many so-called fitness experts are simply not technically prepared to guide you through an effective fat-loss program.

Swimming laps or swimming slow for a certain number of minutes is not as effective as walking for burning body fat. In fact, swimming laps in a pool is a poor way to lose fat weight when compared to walking. Swimming produces about half the fat loss as an equivalent amount of walking. I'm always surprised when some weight-loss amateurs advise that swimming is as good as any other exercise just because it's aerobic. Again, swimming can be beneficial to your health and fitness level, but it's not really effective for losing fat weight.

If you can find the time and the place to swim or take an aerobics class, chances are you can find the time to walk. Paced walking, using our Body Contouring schedules, will get you a very pleasing and very definite result. It works better, doesn't require special clothing or equipment (except good shoes and a supportive bra), and doesn't require you to exhaust yourself. Also, you don't have to know how to swim or dance!

Many new moms find it difficult to go to a health club or gym. The time required to get ready, make plans (and bottles) for the baby, drive to the club, work out and drive back home is enormous. Think of the difference between doing that or simply walking on your treadmill at home while your baby is sleeping, or going for an outdoor walk while someone else watches your baby. And as we've said, walking is better for losing fat than traditional workouts anyway.

One of our clients, Teri, said that she was finally able to stick to her exercise program since she began walking at home. She had been driving to a local health club, but frequently missed her workouts, because she didn't feel like driving or she just didn't feel like getting "dressed up" to go. She said, "I didn't look so great during those first few weeks after my baby was born, and it took a lot of effort to make myself look presentable. Some days, it was just too much trouble—so I stayed home. Now it's a breeze because it's much more convenient, and I can exercise more consistently at home!"

Daily Fat Record

ON THE BOTTOM of each weekly walking schedule (included in Appendix 1 near the back of this book) is a space for you to record your "Dietary Fat Intake." We do not believe "dieting" is beneficial or necessary for you to lose body fat. It's much more important and more effective to first identify and then reduce the excess fat in your diet. A great way to do that is to simply write down the foods you eat during the day that you believe have fat in them. At the end of the week, you have a record of your fat intake. This gives you a good view of your "eating habits." (Check the chapter on the Five Fat Groups to help you identify the sources of fattening foods.) By reviewing your "problem foods," you can gradually reduce the amounts you eat. This easy "daily fat record" method has been extremely popular and effective for participants in our Body Contouring Program.

Look on the bottom of each weekly walking schedule in the Basic Program for your daily "Fat Record" space. Continue to do the Kegals and lower-extremity exercises in the Pre-Conditioning Program from chapter 5.

THE ADVANCED BODY ■ CONTOURING PROGRAM

WHEN YOU HAVE COMPLETED THE SIX-WEEK BASIC PROGRAM, you might wish to accelerate the fat-burning effect in your body. If you faithfully followed the walking schedules we recommended, two critical things have happened inside your body. First, your fat cells have become much better at releasing the fat stored inside of them, and secondly, your muscles have become better at burning fat. These two changes will now allow you to benefit from some additional exercises. We call these "fast-pace exercises" and "booster exercises."

FAST-PACE EXERCISES

PLEASE LOOK AT THE WEEK 7 WALKING SCHEDULE (this is the first week of the Advanced Program). Notice we have added a column called "Fast Pace at 30 min." Look at Day 4 and observe 2x2 min. in parenthesis. This means that on Day 4 of this week you will add some "fast-paced walking" to your normal session.

The Day 4 schedule goes like this: You begin walking just as you did in the "Basic Program." However, when you get to the 30-minute mark you will increase your steps from 25-29 per 15 seconds, to 35 or more per 15 seconds. You will maintain 35 steps or more for two minutes and then slow back down to 25-29 steps again (moderate pace). Stay at your moderate pace for two minutes and then walk "fast" again for two minutes. Then return back to your moderate pace and maintain until your 60 minutes are completed.

The (2x2 min.) means walk at a fast pace for two minutes followed by two minutes at the recommended pace and repeat. You are doing the fast pace part two times, for two minutes, with two minutes of slower walking in between.

These short two-minute intervals help provide a stimulating effect on your fat-burning metabolism. However, as I've mentioned before, do not attempt these until you have completed the six-week "Basic Program" schedule. As always, if you feel any pain, discomfort, or unusual symptoms, stop exercising and call your doctor.

BOOSTER EXERCISES

WE'VE ADDED TWO "BOOSTER EXERCISES" to your program to shape and tone your muscles even more: 1) abdominal crunches; and 2) modified push-ups. These exercises also help accelerate fat burning in your body.

Look at the Week 7 walking schedule (Appendix 1) and you'll see a schedule for the two booster exercises. Under the Day column, notice that these exercises are to be performed on Day 1, Day 3, and Day 6 of the week. Ten abdominal crunches are to be completed two times.

To properly perform an abdominal crunch, lie on your back with both knees bent. Place your hands at your side and slowly raise your head and upper body about three to five inches off the floor by contracting your abdominal muscles. Then slowly lower your head back to the floor. Do this ten times and then rest for one minute and repeat.

To properly perform a modified push-up, stand about twelve to twenty-four inches from a wall. Place your hands on the wall and lower yourself toward the wall, bending your arms, then push away from the wall, keeping your back straight. You should feel some tension in your chest and arm muscles. You also can get on your hands and knees (knees should be resting on a pillow or mat), keep your back straight, bend your arms—thus lowering your body toward the floor—and push yourself back up. In Week 7 do five repetitions of either wall push-ups or floor push-ups.

Another option for gaining upper body strength is to use the baby. When your baby is old enough to support her own head, you can lie on the floor with the baby facing you, her body resting on your chest and stomach. Grasp the baby securely and lift her above your body until your arms are almost straight. Then lower the baby and lift her again. Do the same number of repetitions as prescribed for the other modified push-ups. If you do these 'baby' lifts regularly, your upper body will get stronger and stronger as the baby gets heavier.

At the completion of the Advanced Program, you will have all the knowledge and experience you need to keep the fat off of and out of your body. Use any of the Advanced Program walking schedules to keep your program going. You know your body better than anyone else, so you may wish to design your own program!

Why Diets Don't Work

Dieting is an ill-conceived concept. It produces short-term weight loss at best. Normally, very little of the weight lost by dieting is actually fat. To make matters worse, there is always a negative pay-back with dieting, because when the diet stops, all the weight comes back.

Because diets always come to an end, the weight always comes back—and with a vengeance! There's really no way diets can work. The whole concept of dieting misses the point. Most of the extra pounds we carry around were not produced only by eating too many calories. Most of the extra pounds were the result of too little exercise and too many "fat" calories. Yet 80 percent of the American population believes that "dieting" by restricting calories is the best way to lose weight.

Losing weight by severely reducing calories is not a good way to lose body fat. An example is the anorexic female who often "diets down" to only seventy-five or eighty pounds by eating less than four hundred calories a day. The sad fact is that although she might be very thin, her body-fat percentage can be very high, many times above 30 percent. By comparison, the average woman, ten to fifteen pounds overweight, is typically under 30 percent fat. Strict low-calorie diets don't help you lose body fat. If your caloric intake is extremely low, your metabolism slows down. If your metabolism slows down, your body burns calories at a slower rate. And if you continue restricting calories, your fat cells become more efficient at storing and holding on to fat. That's what we're trying to avoid! Your body slows down to compensate for the lack of fuel. After all, you now have fewer calories to provide energy for your body.

Something has got to give. Your energy levels drop, you become moody, you don't feel good, and your appearance suffers. Everything starts to fall apart. As humans, we can only tolerate this type of energy deprivation for so long. That's why most diets last for only one, two or four weeks. We just can't take it any longer.

YO-YO IS A NO-NO

IT'S WORSE TO LOSE TEN POUNDS and gain it back than to never lose the weight in the first place. You've heard the term, "yo-yo" dieting. That's where you diet and lose ten pounds. Now satisfied with your ten-pound weight loss, you stop dieting. Within a few weeks you gain the ten pounds back. Then you go back on a diet to lose ten pounds. This up and down, yo-yo weight cycling is not only damaging to your health, it's damaging to your appearance, because it makes you fatter.

Have you ever known someone who has lost weight, but still doesn't look very shapely? I heard a woman in her early thirties proudly announce to a group of her friends that she had recently lost twenty pounds. Then she said, "I weigh the same as I did in high school!"

Behind this woman's back someone else noted, "She sure didn't look the same!" Why didn't she? After all, she weighed the same. The answer is that the weight is not in the same places as it was before. It's distributed differently. What caused this change? How could weight shift? Did muscle turn to fat?

By dieting (restricting calories and not exercising), the weight you lose is not all fat. In fact, if you diet to lose ten pounds, only about three pounds of fat is actually lost. The remaining seven pounds is comprised of water, muscle, and sometimes even the minerals from your bones. When you stop dieting, you gain back the ten pounds. Can you predict the composition of those ten pounds? You guessed it! More fat is regained than was lost, many times twice as much. That means six pounds of fat are regained along with four pounds of water and muscle. Let's face it; fat on your body just doesn't look the same as lean, tight muscle. No matter how little you weigh, a high percentage of body fat will likely leave you feeling dissatisfied with your appearance.

Many women go through this yo-yo cycle numerous times. Each cycle adds more fat to your body. Look at the effect of three cycles of losing ten pounds and then gaining it back. In this example, our test subject Barbie has a starting weight of 120 pounds and a body-fat content of 21 percent (this means that 21 percent of her total body weight is fat). Twenty-one percent of 120 pounds means she has twenty-five pounds of fat in her body. That's a pretty good level for both health and appearance—certainly within acceptable limits.

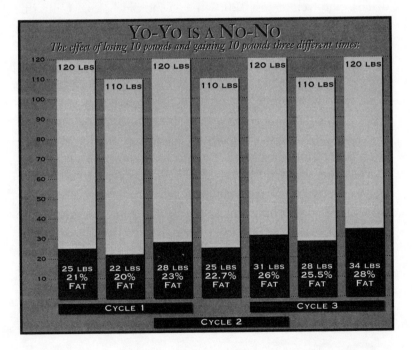

However, summer vacation is only two weeks away and Barbie decides to lose ten pounds to impress her husband, Ken. Lately, Ken has been focusing most of his attention on perfecting a new and improved hair spray for men. This has left Barbie feeling a bit neglected. But losing ten pounds will surely turn his head and his attention back to her. So Barbie diets and loses ten pounds in two weeks. She now weighs a trim 110 pounds (only three of those ten pounds lost are fat; the rest is muscle and water). Her body-fat percentage also drops to 20 percent. Not too bad so far.

The beach trip is a success, and all is well until they get back home. Ken returns to his fascination with hair spray and Barbie is depressed. Why can't he be like other men—insensitive in normal ways? Why can't he just be obsessed with sports? With thoughts like this going through her head, Barbie stops dieting and gains the ten pounds back. This time, though, six pounds of fat are gained back (note: she only lost three pounds of fat). She weighs just 120, same as she did before. Only this time she has more fat. Now her body is 23 percent fat. You can see by the example that each time she loses then gains ten pounds, she gets fatter and fatter. (Personal note to Ken: You are contributing to Barbie's weight gain. Please refer to chapter 11.)

There is another, less obvious reason why this yo-yo pattern is damaging your health and appearance. Each time you lose weight by restricting calories, it becomes harder and harder for you to lose fat weight the next time you try. Your fat cells become sluggish, and there is very little stimulation of lipolytic enzyme production (enzymes that help to release fat from the fat cells). And you have lost some muscle, too. When you lose muscle, your metabolism slows down. On the other hand, active muscle tissue generates heat, driving up metabolism. When your metabolism is increased, you burn more calories, including fat, even while resting!

FINAL THOUGHTS ON DIETS

WHEN YOU MAKE DRASTIC CHANGES in your eating habits, everyone around you suffers, including you. Most women do not need a calorie-restricted diet. They need a fine-tuned eating plan—a set of guidelines to follow for a long time. Any diet or nutritional plan should aim first at improving your health. Then in combination with a well-designed exercise program, it should assist in controlling your weight and contribute positively to your overall appearance. Don't be fooled by the promise of quick weight loss or some unexplained magical effect. If it sounds too good to be true, it probably is!

16

An Eating Plan that Works

*I*t's time to adjust your eating habits to improve your health and get the kind of real weight loss that creates a more contoured appearance. Consistent effort over time is required to achieve the results you want. The good news is that the effort required to get good results is not that hard. However, the effort must be consistent, and certain guidelines must be followed. Look at the following list of eating guidelines. These guidelines will help you develop an approach to eating, not a strict, rigid, boring, and oftentimes, complicated "diet."

- Eat only the foods you like.

- Learn which of the foods you like are healthy.

- Don't avoid foods you love.

- Change eating habits slowly—no drastic changes!

- Don't eat foods you dislike.

- Gradually learn to like more healthy foods.

- Don't rely on willpower alone. Work on changing the way you think about food.

- Don't fast, and don't crash diet!

These eating guidelines promote an eating philosophy rather than a diet. I'm sure there are other useful guidelines. I encourage you to use whatever methods you find to be helpful and healthy.

It's really simple to change a habit or to adopt a new one if you have the correct instructions. If you would like to be successful at improving your eating habits for the better, you might wish to use the following strategies:

FIVE SUCCESS STRATEGIES FOR CHANGING HABITS

- Decide to change because you want to, not because someone else wants you to.

- Find good, accurate information and believe in it. This book is a good start.

- Develop a plan and a realistic timetable.

- Get started—take action. Don't wait until you have it all figured out. Start now and you will benefit sooner. Start now before you lose desire and motivation.

- Don't stop—don't give up until you get what you want. It's okay to modify your plan and to suffer a few setbacks. Remember, don't accept failure. With each setback, you learn something—keep trying.

Now, let's go back to our eight eating guidelines, and examine them in more detail.

1 Only eat foods you like.

That's what most people end up doing anyway. Over your lifetime, you probably eat only foods that you like. Why punish ourselves? One of my weight-loss clients explained to me that she only liked fattening foods. But as I explored her food likes and dislikes, I discovered that she actually liked many foods that were relatively low in fat. Over the past few years, however, she had developed a pattern of eating mostly high-fat foods. She had really chosen to eat this way out of convenience. She worked full time and had two school-aged children and a husband. Her family ate a lot of fast food and at home everyone ate pizza, hot dogs, and other high-fat foods at least three days a week.

Her eating patterns and those of her family members had become habits—bad eating habits. Poor eating habits are difficult to break. First realize that these habits are harmful (damaging to your health and your waistline!). Then decide to break these high-fat eating habits. How? One way is to think about all the healthy, low-fat foods you enjoy eating and begin to work more of these into your diet.

2 Learn which of the foods that you like are healthy.

Let's say that you like about one hundred different kinds of foods. Out of these one hundred foods you find that about seventy to eighty could be healthy if they were prepared or used properly. You could eat them baked instead of fried, select lower fat varieties, or eat lower amounts at one time. It might be that you're eating healthy foods, but in an unhealthy way.

When I was in graduate school a few years ago, I went to a new restaurant with a group of friends. Included on the menu was a "health food" section that was promoted for the "health conscious" consumer. Appetizers included cauliflower, broccoli, mushrooms, and zucchini—all of which are good, healthy choices. However, each of these "health foods" was deep-fried in oil. The chef had taken a perfectly healthy low-fat food and created a high-fat lump of hot grease! That's an example of a "good" food prepared in an unhealthy way.

We asked the waiter if we could get any of these items baked or raw. In both cases, the answer was no. He then told us somewhat proudly that although these foods were fried, only 100 percent vegetable oil was used, and there was no cholesterol in them. Who cares? Vegetable oil is still 100 percent fat, and it has exactly the same amount of calories as lard, butter, or any other type of cooking oil—it's still 100 percent fattening.

If you want to eat healthy foods, make sure the food is prepared in a healthy way–frying is not an option if you want to reduce fat in your diet and in your body!!

3 Don't avoid foods you love.

There are some foods you just can't do without. So, you hate the thought of not getting to eat these foods anymore, right? You might know that a particular food is high in fat, but it really doesn't matter—you must have it! Should you avoid those foods? Absolutely not! Avoiding foods you love creates a feeling of deprivation and loss. Don't deprive yourself of something you love. Just use good judgment, common sense, and a little self-discipline.

You likely will increase your food cravings when you decide never again to eat a food you love. When a craving can no longer be controlled, you might even binge and that can throw you way off track. Don't deprive yourself completely. Instead, reduce the amount of these foods you eat and reduce how often you eat them. If you eat a dozen donuts two times a week, reduce your portion to six donuts twice a week. That done, you will have reduced your fat intake from donuts by 50 percent. Later, reduce your intake of donuts to once a week instead of twice a week, another 50-percent reduction. After a while, your donut consumption might fade even more as you realize that such a high-fat splurge is contradictory to your goal of losing weight. It's okay to give yourself the freedom to eat donuts, but monitor how often and how much you eat.

4 Change eating habits slowly—no drastic changes.

It's not very easy or smart to drastically change your eating habits. Psychologically, it's not very smart because you are upsetting or uprooting a habit. You also start up the "craving" monster. But the real problem is how it affects you physically. Your body does not respond well to sudden change. It needs time to adapt and respond positively to change.

Think about this example. What would happen if I asked you to get up at 4:00 A.M. and run five miles as hard as possible? When you finish, you are to work out with heavy weights for an hour, and then knock out a sixty-mile bike ride. When you complete the bike ride, you are then instructed to run five more miles. Just thinking about this challenge ought to be enough to exhaust you. For most people, that would be a huge challenge. The physical demand on your body would be tremendous. You would probably not be able to complete such a demanding regimen unless you were properly trained. With gradual training, you could possibly do it; your body could adapt and respond.

Changing eating habits also takes time. Your body has to be trained to not crave high-fat foods. Just as a baby is weaned off mother's milk, you must wean yourself off fat. There are two good reasons to gradually reduce fat in your diet:

■ Your taste buds slowly readjust to provide more pleasurable sensations from other low-fat foods; and

■ Fat cravings are reduced.

As you successfully wean yourself from fat, you will learn to really enjoy the taste of low-fat foods. In our program, weaning means reducing your fat intake to no more than twenty percent of your total daily calories.

5 Don't eat foods you don't like.

My favorite high school English teacher told us not to use double negatives such as, "Don't eat foods you don't like." I understand the reasoning behind that grammatical principle—to avoid confusing your intended meaning. If you try to force yourself to eat foods you don't like, guess what? You're on a diet! And that's a double negative—you slow down your metabolism and you store fat easier.

Forcing down foods you don't really like is only a quick fix at best. After all, how long are you going to put up with something you don't like? Not very long. Think about a diet you tried one or two years ago. Are you still on it? Probably not. Most people do not stay on a diet that requires them to eat foods they didn't choose and might not even like.

Remember when you were very young and someone tried to force you to eat something you didn't like? It might have been a family rule to clean your plate before you could get up from the dinner table. "Eat your vegetables, then you can go outside and play."

As a child, you might have been very creative. Disguising food was an art. Rearranging and hiding broccoli under mashed potatoes, or stuffing napkins and pockets with Brussels sprouts and carrots became a challenge. So you probably never enjoyed eating foods you didn't think tasted good. There's no need to force yourself now. However, there is a trick to healthier eating—you can gradually learn to enjoy some of the foods you didn't like before.

6 Gradually learn to like more healthy foods.

This is not as hard as it seems. Things have changed since you last tried those awful-tasting foods. The most important change is your commitment to achieving your weight and appearance goals. If you have truly decided that you will stick with this program, you have taken a giant step—a very necessary step. And you have dramatically increased your chances of getting the results you want. If you have the desire, then your outlook on food is changing.

Sure, you might love great-tasting desserts and other special dishes prepared just to tickle your taste buds. But as you think more and more about your goal (to permanently trim, shape, and lose weight), high-calorie or high-fat foods will become less and less appealing. They still taste good, but you will develop a faster shut-off switch. After a few bites, you will become satisfied and stop eating before any weight damage is done. Immediately, you realize two important benefits:

■ You didn't deprive yourself of something you really like.

■ You didn't eat too much of it.

Your focus gradually shifts from your old ways of eating to a new, healthy way. Most people will begin to experiment with lower-fat recipes and will not give up so easily if each new meal doesn't taste perfect. There are hundreds of low-fat cookbooks that contain excellent recipes that taste great. But you're probably not going to like everything in them. A little experimenting will help you develop a tasty, but low-fat diet.

Resist the idea that you still don't like a certain food that you consider healthy. Give it another shot. Try it again, maybe in a different way. I don't care at all for raw broccoli, but I love it steamed! Have you ever met someone you didn't like at first, but then learned to like him or her? You might only like certain things about that person or you can only stand him or her for a certain amount of time. Yet, you find ways to enjoy being around the person, especially if it benefits you!

Learning to like some foods is similar. Your first impression of a certain food might not be good. It could be because of a preconceived attitude, or the way it was prepared, or the circumstances under which you were exposed to it. Or maybe you just don't like the taste. Whatever the reason, it's always worthwhile to try it again, one more time—you might surprise yourself!

7 Willpower alone does not work.

Although willpower is good to call on in emergency situations, it should not be used routinely to control your eating habits. Willpower normally forces you to either do something you really don't want to, or not do something that you really want to. Willpower actually makes you go against your natural tendencies. And when you continually use willpower to control any of your habits, it's distressing. You are actually causing additional stress in your life. This might seem like a losing situation, but there is an easy way to reduce the amount of willpower you need to break old habits. The best way is to change your attitude. Changing the way you think and feel about a certain food will make it much easier to avoid or resist.

Take Jenny, for instance. She loved high-fat premium vanilla ice cream. She had decided that it would be impossible for her to ever give it up. She explained that she had tried at least ten diets over the previous three years, and the vanilla ice cream had always been her downfall. Because none of the diets would allow real ice cream, she tried to force herself not to eat it. Jenny said that most of the time she would break down within a week and go back to eating her usual pint every night. She also said that the week without her ice cream was pure torture! She used all the willpower she could muster to "force herself not to have something she wanted very badly." But we know that can't go on very long, and it shouldn't.

At 230 pounds, Jenny was desperate for an answer. One simple recommendation changed her life, and her figure. She had to change the way she thought about ice cream. First, she had to believe in her commitment to lose weight and believe that she could really do it. Then she needed to identify those things or foods that were barriers to her weight-loss success.

What were the situations or foods that were keeping her from losing weight? In Jenny's case, it was obvious—hundreds of high-fat calories every day from her ice cream habit. I advised Jenny to think every day about how ice cream was not only making her fat but keeping her fat. She didn't like it at first because I was criticizing her friend (and I used the word fat in reference to her body). My point, although reluctantly accepted by her, was painfully true. Denial was no longer an option. When Jenny acknowledged and accepted this fact about her ice cream habit, her attitude toward ice cream gradually began to change. She still loved the taste, but now she was more aware of the damage it was causing.

Over a period of three months, Jenny weaned herself down to about one small serving each night. Now a pint lasted five days. Jenny said, "Mike, I just don't think I can stop completely, but I'm happy and satisfied with the amount I'm eating." I said, "Congratulations, you have reduced your fat intake from ice cream by 80 percent! And you're happy and obviously not depriving yourself of something you really like—great job!"

During the next six months, Jenny began walking using the Body Contouring Program. She also learned more about the sources of fat in her diet and began to control her eating habits. At the end of the six months, she had lost seventy-five pounds and had tremendously improved her shape and appearance!

If you think about the effects certain foods have on your appearance and health, you can change your eating habits much more easily. The great news is that changes made this way last. You can live with these changes because you are not forcing them on yourself. Instead, you are enjoying the benefits. Here's how to do it:

Decide you will do what it takes.

Don't let anyone or anything stop you.

Give yourself some grace; nobody's perfect.

Identify your high-fat foods.

Tell yourself these high-fat foods are keeping you from your goal.

Tell yourself you're not going to allow these foods to ruin your health and appearance.

Tell that to everyone else, too!

Begin to reduce the portions of these high-fat foods you eat.

Begin to reduce the number of times you eat these foods in a week.

Look for low-fat alternatives; keep trying until you find many you like.

Eat lower-fat foods.

Begin to walk or exercise using our program.

Smile!

■ Keep going!

■ Great job!

7 Don't Fast, and Don't Use a Fad Diet.

Fasting means that you eat next to nothing for a few days. Any time your body is deprived of calories, your metabolism slows down and you burn less fat. Also, any weight loss achieved will be mostly water or muscle tissue you need. Only about three pounds of fat will be lost with a ten-pound weight loss using the fasting method. Don't bother, because as soon as you do resume eating, your undernourished body will automatically try to store as many calories as possible in your cells! You'll gain more fat than you lost every time.

Fad dieting can take several forms. If you notice a diet that promotes or emphasizes eating only one or two special foods only at certain times of the day, that's a fad diet. If a diet suggests eating only high-protein or low-carbohydrate meals, then it's a fad diet. Any diet that uses excessive gimmicks or guarantees miraculous, immediate results is a fad diet. And if a diet forces you to stick to a strict menu or to buy their food, it's a fad diet.

Any diet plan that is not designed to be used for life and doesn't contain balanced nutrition is a fad diet. Don't fall for quick-fix promises. Your nutritional plan should be personal, tasty to you, healthy, and full of high-quality energy. Your personal approach to eating will determine how you select foods that meet your objectives. Choose the best approach for you.

CHAPTER SEVENTEEN

Burn Babyfat, Burn!

Here's what might be the (mis)quote of the century, often spoken so eloquently and expertly by overweight people offering a profound message of explanation:

"I have a slow metabolism."

Many people use this excuse to explain why they're overweight and always tired. They might add that they don't eat very much food and—in fact—eat less food than many of their friends do. You also might be surprised to know that they're telling the truth! They do have a slow metabolism, they really do eat less than their friends, and they really do suffer from a lack of energy. What they don't understand is that they have caused the problem; it didn't just happen. In most cases, a slow metabolism can be reversed by how we eat and how we exercise!

Years ago, I assumed that most overweight people were either lazy or couldn't control their eating habits. Boy, was I wrong! My insensitive attitude was based on the assumption that people who were overweight (overfat) ate much more food than people with "normal" weight. This assumption is simply not true.

In many cases, overweight individuals eat less than trim athletic people. The overweight person who eats fewer calories and does not exercise might not lose much weight at all. The reason is that as you take in fewer and fewer calories, your metabolism slows down more and more. As your metabolism slows down, you burn fewer calories. Although you're eating fewer calories, you might not be using them all. The calories you don't use are stored as fat. It's a downward spiral that results in lower energy levels and very little fat loss.

The good news is that you are in control of your metabolism and you can speed it up if you want to. Most of us want to because we burn more calories all day long and have more energy, too!

▮ SITUATIONS WE CONTROL THAT SLOW METABOLIC RATE

- ▮ Eating a low-calorie diet that's low in carbohydrates

- ▮ Eating too much fat

- ▮ Participating in little or no regular exercise

- ▮ Having unconditioned muscles

- ▮ Having too much body fat

EACH OF THESE FIVE CONDITIONS can be changed with a well-designed exercise and nutrition plan, and consistent effort.

As a new mom, you naturally have added a few pounds of body fat during pregnancy. This happened to provide extra energy (fuel) for you and your baby. After the baby is born, however, the need for all that extra fuel is reduced. The fifteen to thirty pounds of extra fat you added during pregnancy will become permanent if you don't take action.

Have you ever known a shapely woman who gave birth, but still hadn't quite gotten her figure back by the time she became pregnant again? After the second baby, she might be twenty, thirty, or even forty pounds heavier than before she had any children. Then after the third baby she gained twenty more pounds. After three babies, her once shapely body is a distant memory! And it has become much more difficult for her to lose weight and keep it off.

Each time you go through pregnancy and childbirth without getting yourself back in shape, it becomes harder and harder to lose that extra fat weight. The reason is fairly simple; as we get fatter, our metabolism slows down. It becomes more difficult for our body to let go of fat from the fat cells, and it's harder to burn it up!

There is a solution to this metabolic nightmare. Doing two things properly will change your metabolism. Two things will change your appearance, make you feel better, and give you more energy. Of course I'm talking about eating the right way and exercising the right way. For our purpose, the right way means using the methods which produce fat loss and health improvement. Of all the factors that could possibly influence your metabolic rate, exercise and food have the greatest effect.

It's easy to understand that exercise speeds up your metabolism, burns more calories, and helps with weight loss. It might be a little harder to understand how eating more food can also help you lose weight.

When you eat, your metabolic rate increases. Exercise also stimulates your metabolic rate. It's easy to understand that exercise speeds up your metabolism, burns more calories, and helps with weight loss. It might be a little harder to understand how eating more food can also help you lose weight.

I get challenged on this point many times each year. Recently, I was teaching a university health class of about sixty students. I was working through a lecture on nutrition when I mentioned that many overweight people could benefit by eating more food, not less. Immediately, five or six hands went up. I acknowledged one student who began by saying that I had reversed the statement I had just made. She said, "Dr. Trexler, I think you just said something backward. You said that many overweight people should eat more food to help them lose weight." I said, "Thank you for being so alert, but what I said is correct."

Many overweight people can eat more food if they reduce foods that are high in fat and add foods loaded with carbohydrates. Here's how it works: Fats contain nine calories per gram. Carbohydrates contain only four calories per gram. So for every gram of fat you eliminate in your diet, you could add back twice as much carbohydrate and still save one calorie. (Reduce nine calories of fat, add back four calories twice equals eight calories of carbohydrates.) You can eat more food, if you make the right selections.

To people who complain that they have a slow metabolism, I offer this advice, "Eat well and move!" Imagine yourself driving down the road in your car. You're driving at about twenty miles per hour and you say to yourself, "I have a slow car." Is this really true, or are you causing your car to go slow? Can you change this situation? Yes, of course! How can you speed up your car? Just push the gas pedal; the car goes faster and you're burning more fuel. Your body will do the same if you will just keep it moving (you'll burn more fuel, too!).

A key point here is that your car will not go faster or even move at all if there is no fuel in the tank. Your body won't, either. You must eat well to put fuel into your muscles. The fuel your muscles need comes from carbohydrates. Now you have the energy to fuel your fat-burning fire. Does this make sense? It might not at first, especially if you haven't heard this before. When all is said and done, it boils down to this: You need carbohydrates in your system to help burn fat. Your body is kind of like your car. So how do you make it go faster? Put some fuel in the tank and step on the gas!

■ OTHER FACTORS AFFECTING METABOLISM

DID YOU KNOW that just being overweight (overfat) slows down your metabolism? This means that stored fat does not contribute very much to your metabolic rate unless it leaves the fat cell and is burned. On the other hand, muscle is highly active. Your muscles are your body's engines. Muscles allow us to move, and they produce heat by burning the fuel—carbohydrate and fat—that's stored in our bodies. Exercise that helps lower body fat increases your metabolism.

You might have heard the theory about how aging slows down your metabolism. Well, it's not really the process of aging that slows you down; it's the habits that often accompany aging that slow us down. Normally, as we age, we become less and less active. As we become less active, our body composition changes from more muscle to less muscle and from less fat to more fat. Since we have less "active" muscle, as we get older and more "inactive" fat, our metabolic rate slows down. But it doesn't have to be that way. If you work at maintaining your muscles and not getting fatter, you can put the brakes on this "old age" slow-down and even halt many aspects of the aging process.

PREGNANCY

BEING PREGNANT increases your metabolic rate by as much as 50 percent above normal. After all, you're growing a baby inside you, and that takes a lot of energy and nourishment. However, your body happens to be very efficient at storing extra food, just in case food becomes scarce later. Although your metabolism is higher, so is your appetite. As a result, you gain extra weight. After your baby is born, the extra weight you're left with is mostly fat, although some is fluid, blood, swollen uterus, and larger leg muscles. The extra fat weight is truly babyfat, because you wouldn't have gained it if it wasn't for the baby!

More than 70 percent of the women today who are over-weight and have had babies are overweight because they had babies! Not only do you have to grow the baby for nine months and go through labor and delivery, you're also left with a body that has fifteen to thirty extra pounds to lose. It doesn't seem like a fair reward for what you just went through. On a more positive note, your body is primed and ready for a high-quality exercise and nutrition program. You just completed nine months of training, carrying all that extra pregnancy weight around. Because you lost fifteen or so pounds with delivery, you now have less weight to carry, but with the same amount of muscle. It's easier to walk and your body requires less food, even if you are breast-feeding.

■ BREAST-FEEDING

IF YOU ARE BREAST-FEEDING, your body burns more calories every day so as to produce milk. It's fairly common to expect an additional 400 to 500 calories per day to be required for adequate milk production. The fallacy is that many women eat more than the extra 400 calories they need. Many women also ignore the fact that their bodies have prepared them in advance with vast energy reserves for the purpose of breast-feeding.

■ ■ ■ ■ ■ ■ ■
*B*reast-feeding does increase metabolism and breast-feeding moms need additional calories every day.

Remember the extra fat weight you're left with after your baby is born? Let's say you have an extra fifteen pounds of fat after the birth of your baby. There are 3,500 calories in one pound of fat. Multiplying 3,500 calories times 15 pounds equals 52,500. That's right—52,500 calories. Remember, we said you need 400 extra calories per day to provide energy for your body to produce enough milk for your baby. If you have an extra 52,500 calories stored and you use 400 each day, it would take 131 days to use them up. The net result (theoretically) would be that you would only lose the extra 15 pounds you gained during pregnancy. This might explain why so many women stay fat even if they breast-feed. (They eat too many fat calories.)

Breast-feeding does increase metabolism, and breast-feeding moms need additional calories every day. But nature has already provided much of the needed calories in the form of stored fat. Some new moms even eat more than they need and not only fail to lose the pregnancy weight, but also add on some more! I once interviewed a woman named Janet about her weight problem. Janet was about five-foot-five and 175 pounds. She said, "It's not my fault for being overweight, because I breast-fed my little boy for one solid year, and of course I had to eat more food to provide him with the nourishment he needed. And it was basically a sacrifice on my part."

I asked, "How much did you weigh when you first started breast-feeding?"

"Oh, about 140, I guess," she replied.

Then I paused. I observed a change in her defensive expression as she realized her situation. She had been eating above and beyond what she and her little boy needed. The extra calories were converted to fat and stored in the fat cells.

"It's just so confusing," she continued. "Everyone told me to eat more since I was breast-feeding, and I guess I just didn't make the connection. I wanted to make sure my baby got all the nourishment he needed."

That is certainly the goal of breast-feeding—to insure that your baby gets the best nutrition possible. However, if you are gaining weight while breast-feeding, you might wish to check the volume of food you're eating. Most of the time correcting a high-calorie diet involves reducing high-fat foods. In Janet's case we discovered she was eating too much high-fat breakfast meat. When she eliminated sausage from her diet, her weight stabilized and then went down. Not only did her weight improve, but her metabolism increased, and her risks for heart disease and cancer went down! No major diet changes here; just one small modification made the difference.

One word of encouragement to breast-feeding moms: The quality of your diet is more important than the quantity. Your milk-producing glands can produce very high-quality milk if you follow a few important guidelines:

Special Recommendations for Lactating Women[10]

■ Avoid diets and medication that promise rapid weight loss.

■ Eat a wide variety of breads and cereal grains, fruits, vegetables, milk products, and meats or meat alternates each day.

---

[10]Subcommittee for a Clinical Application Guide Committee on Nutritional States During Pregnancy and Lactation. *Nutrition During Pregnancy and Lactation: An Implementation Guide.* Food and Nutrition Board, Institute of Medicine, National Academy of Sciences. (National Academy Press: Washington, D.C., 1992)

■ Take three or more servings of milk products daily.

■ Make a greater effort to eat vitamin-A-rich foods, including carrots, spinach, or other cooked greens, sweet potatoes, and cantaloupe.

■ Be sure to drink when you are thirsty. You will need more fluid than usual.

■ If you drink coffee or other caffeinated beverages, such as Coke, do so in moderation. Two servings daily are unlikely to harm the infant. Caffeine passes into the milk.

18

The Five Fat Groups

Food gives you energy. Indeed, foods containing mostly carbohydrates, such as bread, vegetables, fruits, and cereals, actually help speed up your metabolism and provide you with a steady energy supply. It's important to include plenty of carbohydrates in your diet because they're very active inside your body. On the other hand, fat is not very active and prefers to hibernate inside the cozy walls of your fat cells. That's why it's so difficult to get rid of it. It's locked up half-asleep and has no intention of getting burned!

To achieve the best possible results on your Body Contouring Program, it's extremely important to honestly look at the fat in your diet. Sometimes you can fool yourself into thinking that your diet is low in fat, when in reality it's much too high. For example, my mother once told me she and my dad were on a low-fat diet and had just about eliminated all the sources of fat they used to eat. I was pleased because I had been on her case to start eating better for quite some time. I had been frustrated with their typical American diet—too high in fat! But now they were really trying to cut down. It seemed as though they were making the change. I was watching as my mom made a bowl of low-fat tuna salad for lunch. She was preparing boiled eggs for the salad. I was sure that she would throw away the egg yolks and only use the "whites."

Sure enough, she separated the hard-boiled yolks and put the whites in the bowl. But then incredibly, she ate the yolks. I said, "Mother, what are you doing? You just ate the egg yolks, the fattening part!"

She said, "I just couldn't waste good food."

Shocked, I said, "The yolk is not good food, it's deadly. It's high in saturated fat and it's the most concentrated source of cholesterol on the planet. The good part of an egg is the white part; it's the best source of protein anywhere!"

We both laughed at the irony of this situation. I told her that she was very brave for eating those yolks, and protecting her family from the dangers of fat and cholesterol. But it wasn't necessary to do it at the expense of her own health!

The point is, it's not a good idea to eat high-fat food just to keep from wasting it. There is no value in putting it inside your body; it causes damage, and you just don't need it! After all, where would you rather have all that saturated fat and cholesterol, in the garbage can or in your arteries? In all fairness, my mother is doing a much better job of preparing lower-fat meals. I think she started when I stopped "getting on her case." I wonder what I can complain about next?

Over the past few years, I've noticed that people don't stick with "diets" very well. You probably noticed that, too! It's so hard to follow a diet plan that someone else dreamed up. These "con" artists deprive, rotate, cycle, and confuse everyone, and then sell ineffective and sometimes harmful dieting gimmicks. It's enough to make you sick—and it frequently does.

After observing and listening to literally thousands of people over the past fifteen years, I developed my own approach to eating (not dieting). The concept is simple; start with what you're eating now and begin to adjust it. Gradually fine-tune your diet. Many "diets" say, "Forget about everything you're eating now and only follow our schedule." That approach doesn't work. It's too drastic, too radical, and most people won't follow it for long anyway.

Remember the four basic food groups and how you were taught to eat that way to make sure you got plenty of good nutrition? The result of that approach was that it made everyone fat. It helped make the nation fat, too! The United States Department of Agriculture (USDA) has recently revised its dietary guidelines to reflect a more low-fat and nutritious philosophy. You might be familiar with the Food Pyramid, which recommends more complex carbohydrates and less fat. These are excellent guidelines for weight-conscious and health-conscious people (or for anybody who is conscious).

We should pay special attention to fat in our diet. I'm sure that's a big surprise to you. We might not even be aware of the many common sources of fat in our diets. Fat is everywhere and it sometimes hides from us. So let's grab our detective gear and examine what I call the "Five Fat Groups." This is a system of identifying everyday sources of fat.

Sandy and I have found this system very helpful in reducing fat in our own diets. Weight-loss clients also have found this method to be useful in helping them reduce fat in their diets. If you can identify where the fat is in your food, then you have a better chance of avoiding it. Here are the five fat groups:

- Fried foods

- Oils

- Dairy products

- Meats

- Desserts

Most of the fat in the typical American diet can be found in one of these categories. Let's look at a few examples of each:

1 Fried foods.

Anything fried is automatically high in fat. It doesn't matter if it's fried broccoli, fried potatoes, fried mushrooms, or fried whatever. If it's deep-fried, then it's worse. If it's breaded and then deep-fried, it's even more fattening. The breading soaks up more grease, and that grease is all fat. It's really not too difficult to cut back on fried foods, because frying is just a method of cooking food. You can still eat the same food; it's just cooked another way.

Chicken is a great example. Fried chicken is one of the most fattening foods you can eat. However, if you remove the skin and bake it, then it's one of the lowest! Experiment with herbs, spices, and low-fat sauces to add flavor—if necessary.

2 Oils.

All oils are 100 percent fattening! This statement is sometimes confusing because of all the media advertising about cooking oils. One company advertises that its product is "lower in saturated fat and contains no cholesterol." Another says, "higher in polyunsaturated fat, better for your heart!" Another might say, "contains no animal fat!" Well, from a weight-control standpoint, I say, "Who cares?" No matter what type of oil is in these products, they all are 100 percent fat. And they all will make you equally fat!

It's true that some of these oils might have different effects on your blood-cholesterol levels. Although all vegetable oils (corn, peanut, olive, etc.) are free of any cholesterol, these oils can alter the ratio, or percentage, of the HDL (good) and LDL (bad) cholesterol already inside your body.

You're probably familiar with polyunsaturated cooking oils (corn, safflower, and soybean). When you consume this type of oil, it tends to lower both LDL and HDL cholesterol in your body, and that lowers your total cholesterol. That can be good for your health, but it's not great since HDL, the good stuff, is also lowered.

Monounsaturated oils, found in olive oils and canola oil, tend to lower LDL (bad) and leave HDL (good) alone. Therefore, there is a slightly greater benefit to your health. Saturated oils (animal fat, lard, palm, coconut, etc.) are very damaging to your health, because they cause a rise in total cholesterol levels—especially LDL—and accelerate arteriosclerosis, which clogs up the blood vessels in your heart. So these oils have differing effects on our health; however, they all cause obesity, and that certainly is unhealthy.

Be careful, oil is everywhere! Read labels. If you see the

words "partially hydrogenated vegetable oil," then beware. Not only is it bad for your health, it's terrible for your waistline. Oils like to hide in food. Snack foods, especially chips, crackers, and muffins are normally loaded with cooking oils.

3 Dairy Products.

All regular, or natural, dairy products are high in fat. Whole milk is more than 55 percent fat. And did you know that 2-percent milk is 38 percent fat? That's because the marketing and advertising people decided to mislead us just a little to take the focus off the high-fat content of their product. They report the fat content by weight instead of the percentage of calories.

Twenty percent of the calories in 1 percent milk are fat calories. Think about that for a second. They advertise on the milk carton that the milk in the jug is only 1 percent fat, when in reality 20 percent of the calories in the milk are fat calories. That's like going to a car dealer to buy a new car and the salesman tells you that the car you want is only three thousand. You jump for joy because you think it's a great deal. But when you go in to pay for it, he says that will be twenty-eight thousand dollars. You say, "What? I thought you said it was only three thousand."

"I did, and it's true, it is only three thousand *pounds!*" the salesman says, trying not to laugh through a straight face.

Most of us are not used to thinking in those terms. Knowing the weight of the car is not the most important factor in your decision to buy it or not. Most of the time it's the price; can you afford it? When you are deciding which foods to select for your weight-loss program, it's more important to know the percentage of fat calories in a food item than the weight of the fat.

> *T*wenty percent of the calories in 1 percent milk are fat calories. Think about that for a second. They advertise on the milk carton that the milk in the jug is only 1 percent fat, when in reality 20 percent of the calories in the milk are fat calories.

When choosing milk products, try to get down to at least 1 percent milk (20 percent fat calories), 0.5 percent (10 percent fat calories) or skim, if you can. The lower-fat choices are more nutritious anyway. If you had an eight-ounce glass of whole milk and removed the fat, you would have less than eight ounces left, say seven ounces. Now you have seven ounces of skimmed milk. To make it eight ounces again you would need to add one ounce of skimmed milk to replace the fat. This new eight-ounce glass of milk has more protein, vitamins, and calcium than the whole milk did because it has less fat and more good nutrients. You get all the nutrition and more from the lower-fat dairy products.

Common high-fat dairy items include sweet cream, half and half, sour cream, ice cream, butter, and yogurt. There are good low-fat or nonfat alternatives to all of these products. Choose some that you like.

4 Meats.

Meats are good sources of protein and iron, but are relatively high in fat. But that's just a generalization. You can select high-quality meats that are low in fat and very beneficial to your health. It just takes some careful screening, honest soul-searching, and portion control!

You need to be able to distinguish between high-fat meats and low-fat, healthy meats, and then eat accordingly. All meats should not be lumped into the same "bad" category. Take steak, for instance. Freshly cut red steaks from your supermarket are fairly low in fat. The less marbling they have, the less fat they contain. Marbling is fat, and that's what we're trying to avoid.

Most of our dietary fat problems from meat come from just a few sources: breakfast meats, fast foods, and some sandwich meats. A breakfast meat such as sausage really isn't meat, it's fat! The next time you're at the grocery store, look at some sausage in the meat section. It's not red; it's white, gray, or brown!

Sausage is about 85 percent fat! Sure, you get a little bit of protein, but look at what else you get—a mother lode of saturated, greasy animal fat. And what benefit did you get out of it, other than a very brief moment of taste that disappears as soon as you swallow? But it's going to be with you for a long, long time. Also, as much of it as possible is going to travel straight to your fat cells (hips and thighs first) and stay for an extended vacation. The rest of it will clog up your arteries, raise your cholesterol level, cause colon cancer, and might even make you burp! How disgusting. If you think of sausage this way, it'll be a lot easier to choose to give it up. Bacon and ham are almost as fattening as sausage, and efforts should be made to reduce these so-called meats.

Your fast-food lifestyle might be getting you into dietary trouble. The most popular fast foods also are the most fattening. These include pizza, hot dogs, hamburgers, chicken, fish, Mexican food, and French fries. Pizza is loaded with high-fat cheeses and meats. It's pretty hard to find a low-fat pizza restaurant, so the advice here is to reduce the amount you eat or the number of times per month that you eat pizza.

Hot dogs are like sausage; both are very high in animal fat. They're made about the same way: leftover fat is scraped up and put in a wiener machine or a sausage machine, and out comes a wiener or a sausage link—a fire-roasted hunk of animal fat. What a treat!

It's funny that hamburgers get all the bad press—too high in fat, high in cholesterol, etc. Of all the fast foods I've mentioned, a hamburger with lettuce and tomato is the lowest in fat and could be worked into a low-fat, nutritious diet. While double cheeseburgers, pizza, fried chicken, most chicken sandwiches, and French fries are normally well over 50 percent fat, a hamburger with lettuce and tomato could be as low as 30 percent fat.

Other meats to watch out for include salami, pastrami, kosher-type meats, bologna, and any breaded meats.

So, what's okay? The best is deli-sliced turkey breast (up to 99 percent fat-free), chicken breast (96-98 percent fat-free) and canned tuna in spring water. Also, most grocery stores are now offering diet-lean varieties of hamburger meat (90 percent fat-free). It doesn't take very much to get the nutritional benefits from lean meat—two to three ounces per day is usually enough, even for nursing moms.

5 Desserts.

Have you ever noticed the types of foods that babies crave? Sandy and I were trying to figure out what our little boy, Michael, was saying one day when he was about fourteen months old. The phrase sounded like "mo' budder." Because we were eating breakfast at the time, we looked on the table for clues. He repeated "mo' budder, mo' budder, mo' budder" with increasing urgency in his voice.

We had presented him with almost everything on the table, when he finally stopped and smiled. Sandy had picked up the margarine (we normally call it "butter") to spread on a piece of toast. Michael was satisfied. He wanted more of it. In fact, butter is still his favorite "food." We are born with certain taste preferences. Automatically, we prefer some foods over others. For example, the number-one taste preference for humans is the taste for fat. The number-two taste preference is sugar. Guess what? That equals dessert! That's why it's so hard to find anyone who doesn't like dessert. We are born to love it, so don't feel too guilty when you crave ice cream, chocolate, or cake.

It makes perfect sense that we were created to have these two dominant "tastes." Fat and sugar are the two types of fuel our bodies need for energy. We prefer fat first, because it's loaded with calories, and it can be stored in our body and used as needed. Almost all Americans crave "mo' budder"!

Because food is so easy to get for most Americans, you don't need to store all that extra fat. You get enough food every day to supply your energy needs. Some people get much more than they need. All the extra fuel energy you don't need is taken down to the fat cells and locked up. Just look around; there are a lot of people storing a lot of extra energy (in their hips, thighs, stomach, arms—you get the picture).

Almost all desserts are high in fat. Therefore, they're not really "sweets"—they're fats! Over the years, some people have mistakenly blamed sugar for their weight problems related to eating dessert. Sugar is not the main problem; fat is! Fat makes you fat. To cut down on your fat intake, you don't have to stop eating desserts. Just select or make low-fat alternatives. The goal is to go for the low-fat or nonfat items rather than low sugar items. I've seen some desserts—especially ice cream—that advertise no sugar, made with Nutrasweet. That's a drop in the calorie bucket compared to nonfat ice cream that has sugar in it.

You get a much more dramatic drop in calories and a better metabolic effect if you reduce the fat and worry less about the sugar. After all, sugar in moderate amounts is either loaded or burned in the muscles, and much less is available to be stored in the fat cells.

Some common desserts and snacks high in fat include donuts, cookies, pies, cakes, candy bars, ice cream, bakery-type pastries and muffins, hot fudge cake, whipped cream, and anything that tastes sweet and is greasy.

The Five Fat Groups do not represent a "diet plan," but an approach to eating. The idea is to scan through these high-fat food sources and begin to adjust your food selections. People who are highly committed to improving their figure find that reducing fat in their diet this way gets easier and easier. No depriving or starving—just being smart, and thin!

APPETITE CONTROL ■

THIS IS SUCH AN IMPORTANT SECTION that I'll make a deal with you. If you'll read it carefully, I'll be brief and try to not bore you too much. Deal? Okay. This topic normally stimulates quite a bit of conversation, wonder, and even confusion. Some people say, "When I exercise, I'm always so hungry. I end up eating more and I'm not losing weight. So what's going on?" Good question.

I can sum up how your appetite changes with exercise in three short sentences:

■ When muscle fuel is low or blood glucose (sugar) is low, your appetite is automatically stimulated.

■ Hard exercise uses muscle fuel and lowers blood glucose, therefore, your appetite is stimulated.

■ Low-level exercise burns more fat and less muscle fuel, therefore, appetite is not stimulated.

It's really pretty simple: When you exercise too hard, you burn mostly fuel that's stored in your muscles. Your muscles don't store very much fuel to begin with. So when you use some of it up during harder exercise, your body tries to replace it as quickly as possible. Your brain controls this process. There are two basic ways for fuel to be reloaded into the muscle. One way is for fat to be drawn out of the fat cell, transported to the muscle, and converted into Adenosine Triphosphate (ATP). Now, this would be great since our goal is to drain fat from our cells and burn it up forever! We get smaller, weigh less, and look better. But there's a catch—our fat cells are lazy.

Although the brain sends a message down to the fat cells to get out and go to the muscles, it doesn't happen. They don't want to. Remember, it takes some coaxing, nudging, and patience to get fat out of the cell. So the brain thinks, "I have another option; I'll crank up the old appetite a notch or two!" And since the fat cells wouldn't cooperate, you are almost forced to find something to eat. It's really not fair to place ourselves in this position. Our appetite can increase so much that it's mentally painful to resist eating. Hunger is a "drive."

Here's how to control a raging appetite. First, from a dietary viewpoint, don't starve or deprive yourself. Eat small, controlled portions frequently throughout the day. Resist "snack attacks" for five to ten minutes. Most of the time these "false hunger pangs" disappear. Drink water or eat a very low-calorie snack if you must. Avoid sugar binges. Although moderate amounts of sugar are not harmful, more than two hundred calories per hour can cause a sugar "rebound," causing blood sugar levels to go too low, thereby stimulating appetite again.

From an exercise viewpoint, don't exercise too hard. Low-level, paced walking uses less muscle fuel and conditions your body to release more fat from the cells to provide energy for your muscles. Therefore, the brain doesn't have to force you to go find more food! The bottom line is *hard* exercise stimulates appetite—*easier* exercise does not.

All Calories are not Created Equal

a calorie of fat is not the same as a calorie of carbohydrate. With that, you are hereby introduced to a concept called dietary thermogenesis, which means heat produced from food. You probably know that your body produces heat, because you normally maintain a temperature of 98.6 degrees. Even if you are in a room that's only 72 degrees, your body temperature remains at 98.6 degrees. How does that happen? The answer is simple; The food you eat is converted to fuel, and that fuel is burned by your muscles.

You have a thermostat that works much like the one in your home. When you begin to get too cool, your thermostat causes more fuel to be burned, and you warm up. In the winter, when your house gets too cool, more fuel is burned by the heating system so as to raise the temperature. If you have an electric heating system, your electric power bills go up, too! If you use gas or oil, those bills go up. As it gets colder, more fuel is burned to maintain a comfortable temperature.

When your body is cold, you burn more fuel, too. If you are outside in ten-degree weather with only light clothing, your metabolic rate goes up in an attempt to keep you at 98 degrees. When your metabolic rate goes up, you burn more fuel. (The fuel you burn is measured in calories. A calorie is a measurement of heat produced by burning food.) This is not to suggest that you should run around in ten-degree weather to burn calories. The point I'm making is that the food you eat provides the fuel your body needs to maintain it's 98-degree temperature.

Because our bodies are so good at maintaining a temperature of 98 degrees, why do some people feel cold when others are nice and warm? Have you ever been on a diet and noticed that you were colder than normal? As you restrict your calories, it becomes more difficult to produce enough heat for you to feel warm. Just as if you removed some wood from a fire, it wouldn't produce as much heat. To make the fire hotter, more wood is needed. To make your body warmer, more fuel is needed. Foods rich in carbohydrates are a great source of fuel for your muscles!

Another important aspect of dietary thermogenesis is that all calories are not created equal. There are three types of nutrients that can produce heat (which means there are three nutrients that have calories): fat, carbohydrate and protein. You might already know that fat has nine calories in every gram of weight. Both carbohydrate and protein have four calories in every gram. This means that for the same amount of weight, fat has more than twice the calories as either carbohydrate or protein.

■ ■ ■ ■ ■ ■ ■

The main function of both fat and carbohydrate is to provide energy for you to live and move, just as gasoline is required for your car to start up and move.

I'm often asked to describe how much a gram is. Well, it takes a little over twenty-eight grams to equal one ounce and sixteen ounces to equal one pound. So, if you weighed 120 pounds, you would weigh over fifty-four thousand grams. Exciting, huh? Anyway, let's get back to the three nutrients that contain calories—fat, carbohydrate, and protein.

The main function of both fat and carbohydrate is to provide energy for you to live and move, just as gasoline is required for your car to start up and move. Fat can be stored in great quantities inside your body for your energy needs later on. And it's stored in a variety of interesting places—as you probably observed. It is not uncommon for an average person to store well over one hundred thousand fat calories. Most of this fat is stored in fat cells located just underneath the skin. Thighs, hips, arms, and the abdomen are common areas. We can pinch these body parts and get a good idea of our own problem areas.

Occasionally, a client or student in one of my classes will question the validity of the concept that someone could store that many calories inside his or her body. In response to this question, I show mathematically how a person could easily carry around more than one hundred thousand fat calories.

Example one: Mary weighs 140 pounds and has a body-fat content of 25 percent. How many fat calories does she have in storage? Answer: 140 x .25 = 35 pounds of fat x 3,500 calories per pound = 122,500 fat calories.

Example two: John weighs 240 pounds, but is very athletic and is a member of his college football team. His body-fat content is only 12 percent. How many fat calories does he have in storage? Answer: 240 x .12 = 28.8 pounds of fat x 3,500 calories per pound = 100,800 fat calories.

I once calculated that if our feet would hold out, we could walk five hundred miles on the energy supplied by our stored fat! Therefore, walking two or three miles at a time should be a breeze! It is possible for the average person with one hundred thousand stored fat calories to survive up to three months without eating, as long as they consistently drink water. We have all heard of a political or religious extremist going on a hunger strike for weeks or months, and surviving. If we looked at this starvation idea logically, we would conclude that the "fattest people would live the longest without eating since they have more stored energy. (Caution: never try any starvation diet!)

It's no secret that we can and do store large amounts of fat. On the other hand, carbohydrate is not stored in large amounts in our body. Carbohydrate is stored mostly in the muscles, with the remainder stored in the liver and bloodstream. The storage space for carbohydrate is fairly limited, while fat has a tremendous capacity—fifty to seventy-five billion storage tanks. Most research indicates that, in general, we store less than thirty-five hundred calories in the form of carbohydrate, much less than the one hundred thousand plus fat calories.

The limited carbohydrate storage space presents a problem. Where do the excess carbohydrate calories go? After the storage space in the muscles is filled up, the extra carbohydrate is converted to fat and transported to the fat cell for storage.

Aha, but here is the real dietary secret for weight loss: It takes extra energy to convert carbohydrates to fat. Carbohydrates have to be broken down and reassembled as fat molecules. This process requires work, so calories are burned. Great! By the time these extra carbohydrates are converted and transported to the fat cells, they have burned or lost up to 20 percent of their original calories. This means that if you adjust your food intake to include more carbohydrate and less fat, you get an automatic reduction in calories.

In addition, since there are only about 114 calories per ounce of carbohydrate compared to over 255 calories per ounce of fat, you could eat twice as much carbohydrate rich food and still lose weight. Here is an example of how one type of calorie might not be equal to another type. In this instance, I am comparing carbohydrate calories to fat calories. Compare 2,000 calories of fat to 2,000 calories of carbohydrate.

- Two thousand calories of fat requires very little processing to be stored in your body. You eat the fat and since it is already fat, it can be easily transported to the fat cells. Only about 3 percent of the calories are burned up in this process. Three percent of 2,000 is sixty calories. You lose 60 calories, leaving 1,940 fat calories available for storage.

- Two thousand calories of carbohydrate requires more processing since excess carbohydrates must be converted to fat before being stored in the fat cells. Obviously, it will require more energy to convert a carbohydrate to fat. As we mentioned, it takes up to 20 percent of the total carbohydrate calories to do this. Twenty percent of 2,000 is 400 calories. You lose 400 calories—leaving 1,600 available for storage. You get to eat twice as much carbohydrate as fat and net fewer calories, too! And as an added bonus, your metabolic rate goes up automatically!

Fuel sources, such as gasoline, firewood, coal, kerosene, and fuel oil, burn at different rates. You know that if you poured a gallon of gas on the ground and threw a match on it, it would flame up instantly. It would also burn up very quickly and then go out. If you did the same with a gallon of oil, it would not flame up as fast nor burn as rapidly, but it would burn for a longer time. If you threw a match on a stack of firewood logs, they wouldn't even burn without some care and nurturing, and then only after you helped get the fire going for several minutes. The logs would gradually "catch fire," but would continue to burn for much longer than the gas or oil.

Burning your excess body fat is much like burning a log. It takes a certain technique and a certain amount of time to get started. It also takes a certain technique to keep the fat burning. But once you get it burning, you begin to lose fat weight.

Say you have a stack of firewood burning outside—like a campfire. The logs and sticks should be stacked together in a pile for a campfire to burn. The pile is lit at the bottom by lighting the small sticks or twigs. They catch fire and the fire gradually spreads to the larger logs. After the fire is burning well, it will continue to burn until all the wood is burned up. If you spread out the logs before the fire is all burned up, the fire will slowly go out, leaving some of the wood unburned. For the wood to be burned completely, a certain technique must be used. It must be allowed to stay piled up continuously until it is burned up. When you spread out the wood, the burning stops. You interrupted the process.

Burning fat in your body works much the same way. In order to burn a higher percentage of fat during exercise, you must build your fat-burning fire—much the same way you built your campfire. By starting slowly for several minutes, you can gradually ignite your "very generous" supply of stored fat. However, you must be careful not to interrupt the fat-burning process!

> ■ ■ ■ ■ ■ ■ ■
>
> *In order to burn a higher percentage of fat during exercise, you must build your fat-burning fire— much the same way you built your campfire.*

Here's how to get the fat burning and keep it burning: (For exact time and pace refer to the walking schedules in Appendix 1.)

■ Start slowly for the first five minutes.

■ Gradually increase your walking pace to the twenty-minute mark.

■ Slightly increase your walking pace at the twenty-minute mark, and continue.

Beyond twenty minutes is the true fat-burning zone, especially if you start slow and stay slow.

By walking continuously, you keep the fat burning, and that keeps the fat moving out of storage and into your muscles. Before long you have a trim, shapely, and very pleasing appearance. Nice thought!

How Food Gives You Energy

By now, many of you new moms might be asking yourselves, "Do I really need to know this food and energy stuff?" The answer is yes, because when you have a clear understanding of these principles, you will be even more motivated to follow the Body Contouring Program.

By the way, since I'm the husband of a beautiful and talented wife, and the father of a great little boy, it's really exciting to share this program with you. Every time we share the Body Contouring principles with a new mother, it's a joy to see the success she experiences. We want you to be successful, too, and enjoy the results you achieve.

Learning about health-enhancing factors such as food and energy not only increases your knowledge, but also increases the motivation to achieve what you want as well.

So, here we go. What does an energy system do? An energy system creates and supplies fuel to the muscles so the muscles can contract. When our muscles contract we move—we walk, run, brush our teeth, bend over, pick up the baby, and so on. Our bodies convert the food we eat into fuel (fuel = energy).

There are two basic energy systems that supply fuel to our muscles:

- The Aerobic System

- The Anaerobic System

Dr. Ken Cooper, founder of the prestigious, Dallas-based Cooper Institute, coined the modern-day term "aerobics" back in the late 1960s. He developed a "point system" based on how fast and how far you went during your exercise session. By achieving a certain number of points on a weekly basis, an individual's exercise endurance would increase. (More technically, an individual's cardiorespiratory endurance, measured by oxygen consumption capacity—VO2 max— would likely increase if the aerobics program was consistently followed.)

In the late 1980s, I had the privilege of working as an associate director of continuing education at Dr. Cooper's Institute of Aerobics Research. While working there, I taught exercise and nutrition principles to hundreds of fitness professionals, aerobic dance instructors, and representatives of many government agencies.

It's no secret that many people use some form of aerobic exercise to help stay in shape or lose weight. Many of you have probably taken an aerobics class, where an instructor leads a group through an exercise program with music; or you've used an exercise video at home. During these exercise classes, you are told to keep your heart rate in your target zone. If your heart rate is too low, you are advised to speed up or exercise harder to make your heart beat faster. If your heart rate is too high, you are advised to slow down.

This method of exercising is great for improving the function of your heart and increasing your exercise endurance, but it's not the optimal method for losing or burning body fat! Another form of aerobic exercise taps more directly into your fat reserves. I call this TYPE I aerobic exercise, or fat-burning exercise. We will explore this type of aerobic exercise later in this chapter, but first, let's explore the basis of the aerobic energy system.

THE AEROBIC ENERGY SYSTEM

THE AEROBIC ENERGY SYSTEM provides fuel to the muscles in two basic ways:

■ **Beta oxidation.**

This is a technical term which literally means "fat burning." This form of exercise taps directly into your fat reserves. This energy system is used when Type I exercises are performed. Walking is the best example, although many continuous aerobic exercises can be performed at a slower pace to burn more fat. Our goal is to exercise using this system as much as possible. It takes about twenty minutes of slow, continuous walking to effectively get into this system and burn fat.

■ **Aerobic glycolysis.**

This is a technical term for the breakdown of glycogen in the muscle when oxygen is available. This system provides energy when you exercise in your target heart-rate zone. Running, aerobic dance classes, and stair climbing are common examples. More muscle fuel (glycogen) is used compared to fat.

Since losing extra fat is your goal, we have prepared a program for you that burns more fat with less effort. In fact, we advise you to not get out of breath or exercise too hard! Remember, the harder you exercise, the less fat you burn. The Type I exercises are better for burning fat since they are performed at a slower pace.

We could have titled this book *Bye-Bye Bodyfat.* But since most of the body fat you might have gained is the result of your being pregnant and having a baby, we're going to concentrate on safely getting rid of that extra babyfat.

Some women on our program go beyond just losing their pregnancy weight and fat. Many for the first time in their lives achieve what they consider to be their ideal body shape and ideal weight. The good news is that as you are achieving your desired shape, your health is improving, too. Your health risks are being reduced and you look and feel great!

To actually "burn" excess body fat, you have to create the right conditions in your body. By beginning slowly and gradually increasing your pace, you will increase the rate and percentage of fat released from your fat cells, and increase the rate and percentage of fat burned during exercise. Remember, the only real way to get rid of or reduce the amount of fat in your body is to burn it. This fat must be burned in the muscles.

■ ■ ■ ■ ■ ■

By beginning slowly and gradually increasing your pace, you will increase the rate and percentage of fat released from your fat cells, and increase the rate and percentage of fat burned during exercise.

You can actually train your body to burn greater amounts of fat as you walk. By following the Body Contouring Program, the training happens automatically! You also save more muscle fuel (glycogen), because you are burning more fat. The result is a very pleasing reduction of your body fat and an increase in your energy levels. Why? Because when you burn up most of your muscle fuel (glycogen) by doing more intense exercise, you feel fatigued and tired. But when you exercise slower you "spare" glycogen and burn mostly fat for fuel. This explains how your body-fat levels can go down and your energy levels go up when you exercise more slowly! Let's briefly review the benefits of this program.

■ You exercise at a slower, easier pace.

■ You burn more fat, saving muscle fuel.

■ You lose body fat and have more energy.

■ Your health improves.

All of these benefits occur just by exercising under the right conditions. Paced walking is the most effective way to get these results.

Many people have asked us, "What's the big deal about walking? Why is it better than doing aerobics? Isn't it true that if you get your heart rate up in the target zone and keep it there, you will burn body fat?" In theory, the answer to all three questions is yes. But in reality, not very much fat is burned at that pace.

I know it's confusing because I said you must exercise aerobically to burn fat. Well, there is a catch! Remember when I said that your aerobic energy system provided fuel to your muscles in two basic ways? One way was to burn fuel that's already loaded into the muscle (glycogen). The other way was through a process called beta oxidation, or "fat burning." Think about this for just a second. You know that the faster and harder you exercise, the more muscle fuel you burn. You also know that if you exercise at a fairly slow pace for longer periods of time, you burn more fat. You burn more fat because fat cells "let go" of more so your muscles can use it for fuel. Take your pick—would you rather exercise in a way that burns a higher percentage of fat or a lower percentage of fat? It's a fairly easy choice.

To really understand this concept, it's important to know that all aerobic exercises are not equal in promoting fat loss. Since some of these exercises require more intensity or effort to perform, the aerobic glycolysis energy system is used. These Type II aerobic exercises burn more muscle fuel than fat. All of the Type II aerobic exercises—where you keep your heart rate in a certain target zone—are designed primarily to increase the functional capacity of your heart, lungs, and oxygen-utilization system. But most of these exercises create energy from the fuel in your muscles—not from your fat cells! Let's summarize the two types of aerobic exercise:

TYPE I aerobic exercises are low in intensity (50 to 60 percent of your maximum heart rate) and burn mostly fat for fuel. Beta oxidation produces energy. Types of Type I (fat-burning) aerobic exercise:

- Walking
- Slow biking
- Slow jogging
- Moving slowly with baby

TYPE II aerobic exercises are higher in intensity (60 to 85 percent of your maximum heart rate) and burn mostly fuel that's already loaded inside the muscle (glycogen). Aerobic glycolysis produces energy. Examples of Type II (muscle fuel burning) aerobic exercises:

- Running
- Aerobics classes
- Stair climber
- Swimming
- Rope skipping

If your goal is to lose extra body fat, then choose exercises from the Type I list first. After twelve weeks you can begin to add some Type II exercises if you wish. (Our program emphasizes walking, the best Type I exercise.)

Let's look at why it is more difficult to burn body fat when you exercise too hard. Reba was a twenty-eight-year-old mother of two little girls, and twenty pounds overweight. She wanted to lose weight and had been participating in an aerobics class three times a week for about three months. The aerobics part of the class was only about thirty minutes long, but was of fairly high intensity. The people in the class, including Reba, were normally left huffing and puffing by the end of the thirty minutes.

"It's such a great workout, I can barely drag myself home afterwards," she exclaimed. "But I've only lost five pounds in the three months since I've been going. I feel stronger, but I'm just not losing that much weight."

I wasn't too surprised; after all, she was only burning about two hundred calories during that half hour, and I told her that of those two hundred calories, only about forty were fat calories.

She said, "Yes, but if I burn two hundred calories, they have to come from somewhere, so I should end up losing weight. Won't the fat calories be pulled in to replace those muscle calories I just burned?"

"No, no, not really, Reba," I responded. "In fact, two factors probably prevent you from losing very much body fat when you exercise that way.

"First, when you use muscle fuel, you have less energy and you feel tired. Your blood-sugar levels also are likely to be lower, and this stimulates your appetite. You are very likely to eat more—almost without fail. This is partly responsible for food cravings that many people experience after they exercise too hard. When your muscles are left somewhat depleted, it seems as though you must eat. It's much more difficult to control your appetite when you exercise hard.

"Second, your fat cells have actually become more stubborn during that hard exercise. There's little chance for the fat to get out of the storage cell, get to the muscle, and then be burned! The fat would normally leave its storage tank later, after you have finished and recovered from your exercise. But by then, you've probably already eaten or drank something that makes the need for fat in the muscle unnecessary. The calories you just ate replaced the fuel you burned during the exercise class. The fat didn't have a chance to get out of its cell, go to the muscle and then get burned! This is a pretty unfair situation; you just worked hard, got out of breath, got tired, got hungry, but didn't lose much fat!"

Even if you eat later to replace the calories you burned during a slow walk, you still come out way ahead. That's because you actually burned fat during your walk and not much muscle fuel.

Maybe this explains why many people don't lose weight with hard, strenuous exercise. They might even gain weight, because they stimulate their muscles to grow and they're not allowing their fat to burn. They're just draining and replacing muscle fuel while the extra body fat goes along for the ride!

Even if you eat later to replace the calories you burned during a slow walk, you still come out way ahead. That's because you actually burned fat during your walk and not much muscle fuel. In addition, if you eat a high-carbohydrate meal, 20 percent of the calories are used to digest and process the food. (Remember dietary thermogenesis?) If you didn't overindulge, fewer calories would then remain to be loaded back into the fat cells. You benefited tremendously by knowing how to exercise and how to eat!

Now, how could we change Reba's situation? One way is to get her to slow down and exercise at an easier pace. When I'm talking about the "intensity" of the exercise, I'm really talking about how much effort you're putting out; how hard is it for you? That's intensity! Reba could burn a higher percentage of fat if she changed how fast she was exercising. Reba could burn more fat by exercising at a slower easier pace.

Instead of exercising hard to burn forty fat calories out of a total of two hundred calories, she could exercise slower and longer, and still burn two hundred calories. However, at this slower pace, one hundred twenty fat calories are burned instead of forty!

When Reba exercised very hard, she burned calories quickly—two hundred in thirty minutes. But only about 20 percent of those calories were fat calories. To burn more fat, it takes a little longer. When you walk or exercise more slowly, you burn calories more slowly, so it's important to continue longer. The good news is that you're burning a much higher percentage of fat. If you walk for sixty minutes you could easily burn two hundred calories. But you might burn 60 percent or more of those calories from your fat cells—or one hundred twenty calories. You might have walked longer, but you got to exercise at an easier pace and you burned three times as much fat! This type of exercise approach is appealing to so many people because it's:

■ Easier to do—you can enjoy it instead of dreading it.

■ A good mental break—it helps you change gears from a hectic pace to a more relaxing one.

■ Less strain on your joints, bones, and muscles—you have less soreness and fewer nagging injuries.

And, in addition, low-intensity exercise:

■ Helps you feel and look better—you're fresh, youthful, and energetic.

■ Really improves your health.

■ Really reduces fat!

Sandy and I hope you will complete our Basic and Advanced Body Contouring Programs. The benefits are just too good to pass up!

C H A P T E R T W E N T Y - O N E

Achieving Lifelong Health

ssuming you have recently gone through pregnancy and childbirth, or are about to, you are in need of a special program designed to gently stimulate your metabolism, reshape your body, and protect your health. Our Body Contouring Program is designed to do just that. We emphasize low-level exercise. Low level means easy-to-moderate-paced exercise with no strenuous high-impact, and/or out-of-breath exercises. One of our major concerns for you is to reduce the possibility of any type of injury.

As many as 50 percent of all women participating in aerobic dance exercise classes suffer injuries within the first year of participation. Also, far more injuries occur in people who run, compared to those who walk. But we developed our special walking plan for more than just preventing injury. Walking also burns a higher percentage of fat than either running or aerobics. In essence, walking is superior to running when you consider the benefits of injury prevention and fat burning. This specific walking plan was developed to insure your success at losing fat without pain or discomfort. You also are provided with alternative exercises, just in case you don't like to walk or can't walk due to special circumstances. When you begin to exercise on a regular basis and eat a balanced low-fat diet, several positive benefits occur. The first thing you might notice is that you feel better! You have more energy and you're not tired all the time. The next thing you notice is that you're losing weight and shaping up! But the most important benefit is something that you might not notice at all right away—your long-term health improves dramatically! This is the most important result of this program. Everyone would like to feel better and be sick less often.

Let's look first at some of the physical benefits you can expect by establishing lifelong exercise habits.

■ PHYSICAL BENEFITS OF THE BODY CONTOURING PROGRAM

1 **It increases HDL cholesterol.**

HDL (high density lipoprotein) cholesterol is the "good" cholesterol. The more HDL circulating in your bloodstream, the better. HDL cholesterol reduces the risk for heart disease by helping to "get rid" of LDL cholesterol, the "bad" kind. Women normally have higher HDL levels than men. This might be one reason women have lower rates of heart disease than men do.

It's interesting to note that heart-disease rates in women go up after menopause, when their HDL levels tend to go down. So it's important to keep HDL levels at their highest. The good news is that walking is the best exercise for increasing your HDL cholesterol! If you exercise too hard, HDL levels will not go up and might actually go down.

2 **It promotes a stronger heart and blood vessel system.**

Steady, continuous exercise strengthens your heart and circulatory system. Your heart is a muscle and responds to exercise much like any other muscle does. It gets stronger and it contracts with more force.

Think about someone who wants to make his or her arm muscles stronger. Usually, that person will perform some type of weight-lifting exercise that overloads the muscle. In response to this overload, the muscle gets stronger and in some cases larger, too. However, to make our heart muscle stronger, weight lifting is not needed nor is it recommended. Instead, science has proven that continuous low-level exercise, like walking, works best.

Although your heart is a muscle and can be trained to get stronger, it has a few incredible differences from your other muscles. The most astounding difference is that your heart doesn't get tired as other muscles do. Imagine that. You have something that never gets tired even when you are! A normal healthy heart is an amazing organ; it keeps on beating every second, every minute, day after day, year after year.

An average person has a resting heart rate of about 70 beats every minute. Multiplied by sixty minutes, that's 4,200 heart beats every hour. Next, multiply that times twenty-four hours in a day, and you get 100,800 heart beats every day. Many of us take for granted the miraculous job our heart is doing for us—and without any rest. All of our other muscles get tired fairly easy and stop working until they can rest. Luckily, our heart was designed to keep us alive by never having to stop and rest. Continuous walking for twenty minutes or more strengthens your heart.

3 It burns body fat.

The Body Contouring Program really helps burn away excess body fat. It's hard to contain our enthusiasm for a program that works so well and is so beneficial for our health, too! After all, one of the main points of the book is to show moms how they can shed the extra babyfat they accumulated during pregnancy. Burning excess body fat is a major health benefit. We know that being overweight (especially overfat) causes a variety of health problems: increased risk of heart disease, cancer, stroke, type II diabetes, orthopedic problems, high blood pressure, and so on.

Because our activity program focuses on reducing your body fat, your risk of developing these health problems is reduced. Plus you look better, feel better, and have more energy. One of our clients, Karen, remarked that she had just received the best compliment of her life. Karen is a thirty-seven-year-old mother of three who lost twenty pounds over a three-month period. She also toned and shaped her body using the exercises from our program. She was very pleased with her trim and athletic-looking figure.

Karen soon ran into an old friend from high school. Her friend said, "Karen, is that you? You look twenty-five years old!" Karen was obviously overjoyed with this unexpected compliment. That compliment reinforced Karen's commitment to her exercise program. (If any men are reading this section, you can really boost your mate's confidence and happiness by giving her sincere compliments about how she looks—every day. You, too, will be rewarded!) Feeling good about yourself and receiving compliments might not appear to be health benefits, but they are. Certainly being happy is a positive sign of good health. Losing unwanted body fat is good for you physically and mentally!

4 **It reduces blood pressure and triglycerides.**

It might surprise you to know that walking helps reduce your risk of heart disease even if you have high blood pressure. In a landmark study[11] conducted at the Cooper Institute in Dallas, Dr. Steven Blair and colleagues reported that women could walk the equivalent of two miles in thirty minutes or less, three to four days per week, and reduce premature death rates by 50 percent or more compared to those women who are inactive. This study demonstrated that walking or low-level exercise has a preventive effect against heart disease and even some preventive effect against cancer in women. What a wonderful health benefit!

Many "enlightened" physicians now recommend a walking program for their patients who have moderately high blood pressure. In many cases, these patients never need drugs to control their blood pressure. In fact, many health-care professionals consider a well-designed walking program as the first line of defense against high blood pressure. It's also important to reduce weight and reduce extra retained fluids. If these measures fail to adequately reduce and control elevated blood pressure, the physician might then prescribe blood-pressure medications.

---

[11]Steven N. Blair, P.E.D.; Harold W. Kohl III, M.S.P.H.; Ralph F. Paffenberger, Jr., M.D., Ph. D.; Debra G. Clark, M.S.; Kenneth H. Cooper, M.D., M.P.H.; and Larry W. Gibbons, M.D., M.P.H., "Physical Fitness and All-Cause Mortality: A Prospective Study of Healthy Men and Women," *Journal of the American Medical Association*, November 3, 1989 (American Medical Association: Chicago, Illinois). Vol. 262, No. 17, pp. 2,395-2,401.

Triglyceride is the name for fat that circulates in our blood and is stored in our fat cells. Remember our fifty billion fat cells? Stored inside of each one is a drop of triglyceride. Some people have larger amounts of triglyceride stored in each drop, so they are larger, too! And guess what? That's the fat you're trying to get rid of! Our goal is to get the triglyceride fat out of the fat cells, out of the bloodstream, and into the muscles where it can be burned up forever!

If you have too much triglyceride floating around in your bloodstream, your risk of heart disease is increased. But since most of the triglyceride in your blood comes directly from the food you eat, you can reduce it by eating less fat. And since triglyceride can be burned away if you exercise the right way, you can reduce it even more. You can reduce the amount of triglyceride circulating in your bloodstream by 20 percent or more in less than one week—primarily through reducing dietary fat intake.

5 **It helps digestion and reduces indigestion, gas, and constipation.**

Your digestive system is very efficient at taking whatever you put in your mouth and squeezing out the nutrients your body needs. The sad fact is most people are much less concerned about the quality of fuel they put in their bodies than they are about the fuel they put in their cars. Many times people tend to eat food because of the way it tastes, not because of its nutritional value.

What if you chose fuel for your car by how it smelled, tasted, or looked? Unless you make the correct choices, your car won't run very well. But if you put the right type of fuel in your car, it runs as it should. If you put the right type of fuel in your body, it works well, too. Luckily, your body has a super fueling system! It starts with the digestive system.

Your digestive system is comprised mainly of your mouth and teeth, esophagus (the tube running from mouth to stomach), stomach, small intestines, and large intestines (colon).

Here's how digestion works:

■ Food enters the mouth, where chewing and saliva begin to break down food.

■ The chewed food is swallowed and slides down the esophagus to the stomach.

■ Strong acids in the stomach break down the food further and further; the stomach mixes the food much like a blender or cement mixer.

■ The blended mixture leaves the stomach and passes into the small intestines where most of the food is absorbed into the bloodstream. This is where the carbohydrates, fats, proteins, vitamins and minerals pass through the intestinal wall. Your bloodstream carries these nutrients to all parts of your body.

■ Leftover waste, including fiber, passes into the large intestine and is eliminated from the body through the rectum and anus.

It's a very efficient system. However, we all experience occasional problems with this normally smooth-running process. For women who are either pregnant, or have recently delivered, we have noticed two common problems: 1) indigestion or gas; and 2) constipation. Indigestion and gas occur much more frequently in pregnancy than at any other time. Usually, it's the result of the increased amount of food being consumed which produces a greater volume of gas. Or, it's because the stomach is being squeezed and compressed by a growing and active baby. Since the stomach is forced into a smaller space, indigestion and gas can be reduced by eating smaller amounts of food at one time. Although you will increase the number of times you eat each day, food will move through your body quicker and produce less discomfort.

If your baby is already here, you might be facing another common problem—constipation. Seventy to 80 percent of women in the postpartum period report at least some difficulty with constipation. Regular exercise and balanced, low-fat, high-fiber eating can really help reduce or even eliminate these problems.

Some women rely too heavily on high-fiber cereals or supplements. You can actually cause constipation if you don't drink enough fluids to go along with the fiber. Have you ever noticed what happens to a bowl of high-fiber cereal if you let it sit there for a while? It soaks up all the milk! And it expands. For fiber to work for you, you must drink plenty of fluids to keep the fiber bulk soft and moist. How to stay more regular and avoid constipation:

■ ■ ■ ■ ■ ■

*S*eventy to 80 percent of women in the postpartum period report at least some difficulty with constipation. Regular exercise and balanced, low-fat, high-fiber eating can really help reduce or even eliminate these problems.

- ■ Eat more watery fruits and vegetables (oranges, apples, melons, tomatoes, etc.).

- ■ Eat high-fiber foods.

- ■ Drink more water, especially if you're breast-feeding (eight to twelve eight-ounce glasses a day).

- ■ Monitor caffeine and alcohol intake. Too much can have a diuretic effect.

- ■ Reduce heavy refined foods (high-fat, high-sugar foods contain very little fiber or water.

- ■ Walk as recommended by our program.

As your body adjusts to a regular exercise program and a high quality diet, constipation will likely occur rarely, and might even become a thing of the past!

6 **It increases muscle tone and energy levels.**
Most people don't realize that when they increase their muscle tone, their energy levels go up. Your increased energy is not really the result of your muscles being toned. It's the result

of what you did to make your muscles toned. To get toned muscles from the Body Contouring Program, you have to exercise. Paced walking stimulates your metabolism, reduces body fat, and creates more usable energy for you!

Toned muscles are stronger and more powerful than flabby, out-of-shape muscles, and they are more resistant to injury. Your knees, hips, back, shoulders, and neck are stabilized better with tight, firm muscles. It's no wonder that many physical therapists and exercise specialists recommend abdominal exercises to relieve lower back problems. Strengthening the muscles in the stomach area help support the lower back structure. Stronger toned muscles help prevent strain and injury.

7 It stimulates bone production.

Weight-bearing exercises such as walking help make your bones stronger. This is especially important for women in the child-bearing years. Beyond age thirty-five, bone production in women slows down dramatically. This means that the bones in your hip, pelvis, spine, arms, and legs get weaker as you get older.

You might be aware that pelvic fractures are fairly common in older women, and the complications often lead to death. Since it's difficult to build additional bone strength after age forty, it's important to build as much as possible before then and to hold on to as much as possible afterwards. The harder and stronger your bones are, the less likely they are to break.

There are a few ways to build and maintain more bone strength:

■ **Weight-bearing exercise.**
  Walking is best for lower body; pushing/pulling with light weights or other resistance exercises for upper body is better.

■ **Twelve hundred milligrams of calcium each day.**
  It's best to get calcium from low-fat or skim dairy products since vitamin D found in these products can aid in calcium absorption and fat intake is lowered.

■ **Adequate vitamin C.**

Intake of sixty to two hundred milligrams per day can help calcium get absorbed into the bone. Although the recommended daily allowance for vitamin C is sixty milligrams, you might benefit from a little more if you smoke, lose large amounts of water through urination or sweat, or drink excessive amounts of alcohol. There is no documented need or benefit from large doses of vitamin C.

If you have had a hysterectomy or have gone through menopause, you should speak to your doctor about estrogen therapy to help prevent osteoporosis.

It's great to know that our health will actually improve by following the Body Contouring Program. We all know people who have gotten sick on fad diets, crash diets (that's an appropriate term), or even supervised-fasting diets. If a diet makes you sick, it can't be good for you. And no one wants to stay on a diet forever.

Most of you probably know someone who has been injured by exercising too much or doing the wrong types of exercise. Accidents happen, but most of these exercise injuries occur from a lack of knowledge; not by accident. You don't get thin or healthy by accident, either—it's by design!

THE FIVE DIMENSIONS OF HEALTH ■

TRUE HEALTH HAS MANY DIMENSIONS. In other words, there are many types of health. So far, Sandy has talked a great deal about our emotional health, and I have focused on our physical health. Although these are important areas, there are a few more that also are important to consider.

Over the past few years, I have conducted more than one thousand health-related lectures and presentations in a variety of settings, including: The University Of Arkansas, fitness institutions, state police academies, business and community organizations, and even the Secret Service in Washington, D.C. A common theme I tried to address throughout these health lectures was that health involves five distinct areas (or, as we said, dimensions):

■ physical

■ emotional

■ spiritual

■ intellectual

■ social

Almost all of our experiences here on earth could probably fit into one of these five categories. I've been tempted to add a couple of categories to the list: environmental and financial. But when I really think about it, the environment affects our physical and emotional health, and finances usually affect us emotionally, as well as how we interact on a social level. You might have a different interpretation.

1 **Physical health.**

We've talked a great deal about this area, because it's a major focus of the book. The idea of physical health is to improve your resistance to disease, injury, and premature death. This is accomplished through improvements in strength, endurance, flexibility, energy levels, body fat, and weight. It's also important to:

■ abstain from smoking

■ eat a low-fat, balanced diet
■ use alcohol only in moderation

■ wear seat belts

■ avoid risk-taking behaviors

■ remain in a monogamous sexual relationship

If you do well in these areas, the side effect is an improved appearance—an added bonus for practicing good physical health habits.

2 Emotional health.

Emotional well-being is required if you are to be truly healthy and happy. Emotional health involves balanced and rational thinking, along with an optimistic and stable outlook on life. People who are functioning well in this area express their feelings freely and are able to cope with stress more easily. A hardy or resilient personality increases the stability of emotional health. (Sandy has provided you with a wealth of emotional information in the first nine chapters of this book.)

Spiritual health.

Most people have their own ideas about spirituality. Some believe spiritual matters are only related to certain religions. Actually, spirituality is a part of us all, whether you are religious or not. It is important for your health's sake to have a strong value system that is consistent with your beliefs. Humans desire a sense of belonging and a sense of worth. Having a baby can bring a new, deeper sense of worth.

Also, you need to know and feel that you are valued for who you are, and that you are not alone. Many people are at peace with themselves and those around them due to their faith. Inner turmoil is resolved and a compassionate helping attitude is the result. These peaceful, enlightened people are certainly achieving very high levels of health and well-being.

Intellectual health.

When you are mentally stimulated, your intellectual health improves. If you are a new mom, you know how it feels to be at home all day long with just your baby (or even with other small children). By the end of the day, you need some mental stimulation, some conversation with an adult—any adult!

After our son, Michael, was born, Sandy would often call me at work hinting that she needed to get out of the house and talk to someone. At the time I really didn't understand what she needed. I later realized, with her help, that when I came home I was talking "baby talk" to both Michael and to her. I would say, " How's my big, little baby boy," and then I would play with him and ask Mommy what they did all day. I stayed in the baby talk mode—not only talking baby talk, but centering my part of the conversation on the events surrounding him. Sandy needed some mental stimulation. It took me a while to help provide this for her.

Other signs of good intellectual health include the desire to seek out and understand new information, to feel competent in your ability to solve problems, and to be curious about your world and your surroundings.

5 Social health.

The relationships you establish with others can be the glue that secures and holds together your total health. Starting with your spouse, these relationships often determine how well you function in society. Connection with family and friends, and interacting well with people you come in contact with is a very positive part of your overall health profile. If you are unable to form bonds with other people, you are probably not a very happy or healthy person. Isolation is detrimental to health. However, some people only require a few close bonds to be happy and satisfied in this important area of health.

As you went through the five dimensions of health, were you thinking of how well you're doing in each of these areas? To be truthful, each time I talk or write about this, I feel a little disappointed that I sometimes focus on only one or two areas, often at the expense of the others. However, if you are aware of these five areas and try to improve just a little bit in each one, your overall health will improve.

CHAPTER TWENTY-TWO

Answers to Common Postpartum Questions

Q *This is my first day back from the hospital. My doctor gave me a prescription for pain medication, and my episiotomy is really hurting. But I'm breast-feeding, and I keep thinking the medication might hurt my baby. What do you think?*

A Anything you put into your body is passed on in small amounts to your breast milk, and thus to your baby. Ask your doctor about the medication and remind him or her that you are breast-feeding. If your doctor knows you are breast-feeding, then very likely he or she has given you a pain medication that will not have harmful effects on your baby. Don't be concerned about taking the medication that he prescribes according to his instructions. However, if you still feel uncomfortable taking pain medication, try more conservative measures to relieve your episiotomy pain, such as warm sitz baths, ice packs, and pain-relief spray which can be applied directly on the incision.

Q *Should I still be bleeding? It's been three weeks since my delivery, and I thought the bleeding would have stopped by now.*

A In most cases it is quite normal to experience bleeding at three weeks. Most women have irregular bleeding for up to two months after delivery. However, if your bleeding is unusually heavy, if it is running down the side of your leg even when you're wearing a sanitary napkin, or if it is completely soaking a pad every few minutes, you should consult your physician. Some women bleed every day for six weeks after delivery, and some women experience very little bleeding.

Q *I've stopped producing milk, and it's only been one week since my baby was born. Is that normal?*

A If you are not breast-feeding, it is normal for your milk production to have stopped. If you're trying to breast-feed, immediately consult a lactation specialist to help you determine what the problem is and how to correct it.

Q *When can I travel?*

A In most cases, you can travel when you feel like it. Most significant problems happen within the first week after delivery. To be on the safe side, stay close to home for a week or so. Chances are you won't feel like riding in a car during the first week or so anyway. After that, go when you feel like going.

Q *It's been four weeks since my baby was born, and I'm not bleeding. Can I jog?*

A No! There is virtually no benefit to jogging during the early postpartum period, and there are many risks. Physicians report cases of postpartum patients who were recovering beautifully, yet experienced significant setbacks because they began jogging too soon. Your uterus needs time to heal, and the ligaments which hold it in place must tighten back up. Your joints are more loose after delivery, due to a hormone secreted during pregnancy which allows the baby to pass through the pelvis. That hormone, relaxin, affects all the joints in the body and has been found to remain in your system for about six weeks or more after delivery. Therefore, your knees and ankles are more likely to become injured during this time. Jogging is not recommended for at least six weeks, or until you are completely healed.

Walking is a much better choice. It will help your body heal, help you drop excess fat, keep you in great cardiovascular condition, and will not cause the jarring and trauma experienced while jogging.

Q *Can I do arm weights? It's been four weeks since my delivery.*

A Yes, if you use light weights and breathe during each contraction. Always avoid holding your breath during any exercise. Stick with light weights for another couple of weeks (not more than ten pounds) and exhale as you lift—inhale as you let the weight down.

Q *How can I melt off some pounds?*

A Your best bet is to stick with the Body Contouring Program. The most effective way to lose excess fat after delivery is to practice low-fat eating, combined with the proper form of walking.

Q *Why can't I seem to lose weight? I'm too tired to exercise, but I'm watching my diet carefully and avoiding high-fat foods.*

A It is very difficult to lose excess fat after delivery without walking. The type of walking recommended in the Body Contouring Program causes the excess fat stored in your fat cells to be released and burned up in the muscle. If you will begin walking, you will find that it actually gives you more energy in the long run. Walking relieves stress, promotes better quality sleep, and improves overall health. These are important benefits for anyone—especially for new moms!

Q *How much exercise can I do? It's been three days since my delivery, and I am becoming very anxious about all this excess weight I'm carrying around.*

A We believe that the more you do now, the more you can do in the future. You should begin the Body Contouring Pre-Conditioning Program now. It will gradually help your body to tighten up loose muscles and drop excess fat tissue. With your doctor's consent, the sooner after delivery you begin a safe and effective exercise program, the better off you'll be.

Q *I am breast-feeding. Can I still get pregnant?*

A Yes! This has been proven time and time again. If you are breast-feeding six to eight times a day, your chances of ovulating are less than 5 percent. You should have unprotected sexual intercourse only if you are comfortable with a 5-percent chance of becoming pregnant! Once you begin having regular periods, you have a much higher chance of conceiving. If you don't want to become pregnant, use some form of birth control.

Q *Is it safe to take birth-control pills while I'm breast-feeding? I don't want to get pregnant.*

A Many physicians feel comfortable prescribing low-dose oral contraceptives for women who are breast-feeding. Ask your doctor.

Q *I had a C-section and its been one week. Can I exercise?*

A Yes, as long as you are not experiencing complications, and your doctor says it's okay. Follow the Body Contouring Pre-Conditioning Program and take it easy. If you feel pain, stop. Early exercise is probably the most beneficial thing you can do to enhance your recovery.

Q *Why do I feel so "blue"? I have no reason to be.*

A During the initial postpartum period (the first six weeks), it is normal to feel a little down. You have been through a major physical exertion, you're probably not getting enough high quality, deep sleep, and you are experiencing the stress that comes with having a new baby. Lack of quality sleep is one of the leading causes of postpartum blues. Work it out with your husband or a relative to help you get more sleep. Pump your breasts and trade off night feedings with someone, and take the phone off the hook so you can nap when the baby naps. Learn new ways of managing stress, and exercise—both will help improve the quality of your sleep.

Q *It's been six weeks and it still hurts to have sex. Is that normal?*

A Yes. Many women have discomfort with intercourse for several months after delivery. If you are breast-feeding, the lining of your vagina is thinner and drier—due to hormones associated with breast-feeding. You also might have lingering pain from your episiotomy. Pain also might be caused by being overly tense. Often, women are understandably afraid of intercourse because they are concerned it might damage their newly healed perineum. Once your doctor gives you the go-ahead at your six-week check-up, you can rest assured that your perineum is healed and will not be damaged by intercourse. However, if you're still not comfortable, you might need to give yourself a little more time.

If you want to have sex, try an over-the-counter vaginal lubricant such as K-Y Jelly or Replense. This should relieve most discomfort associated with intercourse. Avoid petroleum-based lubricants such as Vaseline. If you continue to experience problems, or if you feel sharp or unusual pain, consult your doctor.

Q *Will my stretch marks go away?*

A Probably not. Unfortunately, the tendency to get stretch marks—or not to get them—is usually genetic. If you've inherited this trait, you will probably get stretch marks no matter what you do. Controlling the amount of weight gained during pregnancy might minimize the number and severity of stretch marks, but once you have them, they are there to stay. If they are red and dark, they will probably fade to a more silvery color.

Q *I don't want to breast-feed anymore. I've been doing it for six weeks, and I feel guilty about wanting to stop. Will it hurt my baby?*

A There are many benefits associated with breast-feeding. One of the benefits is the transferring of antibodies from mother to baby. This is said to be most critical in the first month or two after the baby is born. So you have provided your baby with a good start.

Many baby formulas provide excellent nutrition for your newborn, even though breast milk has been shown to be the best source of infant nutrition. If you've decided to stop, wean your baby slowly over the next few weeks. This will make the transition more comfortable for you and your baby. Rest assured you can still provide your baby with adequate nourishment. Have your pediatrician recommend an infant formula.

Once you've stopped breast-feeding, continue to increase the closeness and bonding you've already established by holding the baby close when you give him or her a bottle, and by frequently making eye contact, and talking or singing to your baby. An infant should never be left alone to feed from a propped-up bottle.

If you're thinking about quitting because you must return to work, or because you feel that you are "tied down," you might want to consider pumping your breasts for feedings while you are away, and nursing at night, or using an infant formula during the day and continuing to nurse while you are at home in the evenings.

If your reason for wanting to quit is that you are having difficulties with technique or are concerned that your baby is not getting enough milk, consult a lactation specialist. You might simply need some help and support.

Q *It's been six weeks since my daughter was born, and I feel fat. Can I have some diet pills?*

A No. So-called "diet pills" are a poor substitute for following a program to lose fat, and shape and tone your body. Most people who take diet pills have significant rebound (regaining of even more fat than they lost) immediately after they stop taking the pills.

Q *I still feel terrible. I look terrible. I'm not sleeping, and I cry all the time. Can you give me something?*

A There is not a magical pill which can make you feel better when you have postpartum blues. However, there are many things you can do. Get someone to help you with caring for the baby so you can catch up on much-needed sleep. Sleep deprivation is one of the primary causes of postpartum blues. When you are tired, your perceptions are altered. Everything seems worse than it is.

Exercise works wonders in helping you overcome the blues, as does a healthy diet. Remember, feeling blue is normal. You're not crazy, and there is nothing wrong with you. This blue phase is temporary and will pass. Talk about your feelings with your husband or a friend. (If you are having thoughts of harming yourself or your baby, or find yourself unable to function, your condition is more serious than normal postpartum blues and you might require medication. You should seek professional help immediately.)

Q *Will my abdominal muscles go back to normal if I exercise?*

A Yes. If you do appropriate postpartum exercises such as the ones recommended in this book, your abdominal muscles will tighten up and become flat and toned. However, this will not happen without consistent exercise. If you don't do appropriate exercises to strengthen your abdominal muscles, they will remain stretched and weakened.

Q *What can I do about my weight? I gained forty pounds and only lost fifteen. I am breast-feeding.*

A You must make sure you get adequate nutrition for breast-feeding, as recommended in the breast-feeding section of this book (chapter 3). But you can successfully breast-feed your baby without taking in excess fat and without overdoing it on caloric consumption. You need about four to five hundred calories in excess of your normal caloric intake to breast-feed your baby. That means you could eat an extra orange, banana, and a glass of skim milk each day—or you could eat cookies and donuts. Obviously, the fruit and milk is better for the baby, and will allow you to gradually lose your excess fat. You also need to make sure you exercise regularly.

Q *I am ready to stop breast-feeding. How can I stop my milk flow?*

A As you begin to wean your infant, you need to wear a good, support bra twenty-four hours a day. You want to avoid any stimulation of the breasts—even movement during walking. If this does not work, your physician can prescribe medication to stop your milk flow.

Q *One of my breasts has a reddish area on it, and it's very sore. What should I do?*

A Try to keep the breast as empty as possible. Apply heat before and during nursing, and gently massage the area. If it continues to hurt, and you notice red streaks or discharge, or if you experience flu-like symptoms such as fatigue, fever, and achiness, you could have mastitis—an infection in the breast tissue. This infection does not adversely affect your milk and you should continue to breast-feed. Try to rest as much as possible, and continue with warm moist heat and massage the affected area. Consult your physician, as he or she might want to prescribe antibiotics.

Q *There is a lump in one of my breasts. What is it?*

A If the lump has just appeared since you've been breast-feeding, you probably have a clogged milk duct. This condition is simply a plugging of a duct which goes from your nipple to your milk reservoir. Plugged ducts usually occur on the outer quadrant of your breast (area nearest to your arm). Use warm, moist compresses and massage the area. Continue to breast-feed as often as possible—this will help release the plug.

As you feed, try to point the baby's chin toward the plugged area. Massage the area during feedings, applying pressure from the plug to the nipple, and allow the baby to feed on the affected breast first. Remember the saying, "Heat, rest, and an empty breast"? If the lump doesn't go away in a few days, consult your physician.

Q *My breasts keep getting engorged. What can I do?*

A Try to make sure you're emptying your breasts completely when you breast-feed. Wear a supportive bra when you are not breast-feeding. Severe engorgement might be relieved by using ice packs. If you are not breast-feeding, consult your physician. He can give you medication to eliminate milk flow.

Q *I am still having problems with constipation. I've been home from the hospital for two weeks. What should I do?*

A Eat a high-fiber diet and increase your fluid intake. First thing in the morning, before you eat any food, drink a large glass of water, then drink a glass of prune juice, a small glass of lemon juice mixed with water, or eat an orange. Try one of the high-fiber breakfast cereals—such as All Bran or Fiber One. Minimize or avoid substances known to dehydrate, such as caffeine and alcohol. If you still have problems, try a stool softener.

Q *I am having problems with my hemorrhoids. Is there a treatment?*

A The best thing to do is increase fluid intake and fiber in your diet to avoid constipation and straining during bowel movements, and use over-the-counter preparations to relieve discomfort (such as Preparation H). If you continue to have problems, your physician might need to do an examination to see if you have a more serious problem.

Q *I am experiencing a burning sensation when I urinate. Is there something wrong?*

A Probably not. Most women have some discomfort when urinating after they deliver. If you delivered vaginally, you probably had some trauma to your urethra (the opening where urine comes out) and this would cause some pain. If you had a C-section, the discomfort you feel could be related to the catheter inserted during delivery. If you feel a more frequent urge to urinate and pain continues, you could have a urinary tract infection, and you should contact your doctor.

Q *When can my husband and I start having sex? It's been five weeks and I feel ready.*

A If you did not have an episiotomy, many physicians feel comfortable giving the go-ahead for sexual intercourse at about four weeks after delivery—if you feel like it. However, if you had an episiotomy or experienced some degree of tearing, wait until your follow-up visit at six weeks postpartum—and get your doctor's okay.

Q *How long will my episiotomy keep hurting?*

A Most women experience significant discomfort from an episiotomy for two or three days, then the pain begins to decrease in intensity daily for the next two to four weeks. If the pain begins to increase, rather than decrease in intensity—or if you start to notice a foul odor, contact your physician.

Q *Does delivery "stretch out" a woman's hipbones? Will my hips be wider than before, even after I lose this extra weight?*

A No. During the later stages of pregnancy, you might feel like your hipbones are spreading as the baby settles into the birth canal. In order for your baby to be delivered vaginally, his or her head must conform to your pelvis, rather than your pelvis stretching to accommodate the infant's head. If there is some slight pelvic relaxing during delivery, things should go back to normal soon after.

Q *Will my stretched-out, loose skin ever tighten up?*

A Skin is attached to muscle, and as your abdominal muscles tighten up with exercise, your skin should tighten up as well. In some cases, where there has been extreme weight gain, the skin might remain somewhat loose even after the muscles have regained tone.

Q *How long do I have to breast-feed my baby in order to give him the health benefits associated with breast-feeding?*

A The first two months are when the baby is said to gain the most benefit from antibodies transferred from the mother's body. The general benefits of breast-feeding continue well beyond two months, but the first two months are believed to be most advantageous to the baby. However, breast-feeding has been shown to provide a dose-related benefit. In other words, while two months of breast-feeding is very beneficial, twelve months is even more so. The U.S. Surgeon General's goal for American babies is that they be breast-fed for two years to provide maximum benefit. You need to choose, with your partner, what the two of you feel best suits your baby.

Q *Why does my vagina seem so dry when we make love? It's been eight weeks.*

A Again, the hormones associated with breast-feeding cause a woman's ovaries not to produce as much of the normal hormones responsible for lubricating the vagina. Over-the-counter lubricants should alleviate the problem.

Q *Will my vagina ever be back to its normal size? It feels so stretched out during sex.*

A Most women can return to normal size if they do Kegal exercises regularly. That is the only way to restore muscle tone in the vaginal area. Occasionally, separation in muscle structures can result in a permanently loose vagina, and if this is a problem, there are surgical procedures which can correct it.

Q *It has been six weeks since my delivery, and my doctor said it was okay for us to have sex, but I still don't feel like it. Is that normal? My husband sure doesn't think so.*

A Yes. Many factors associated with your sex drive are affected when you have a new baby. Physical healing is just one of those factors. Others include: overcoming the fear that having sex will hurt; fatigue; low self-esteem related to your body image; lack of exercise; and being consumed with caring for the baby. Communicate how you're feeling to your husband. If you can both relax, your sex life should resume naturally in a reasonable amount of time. All women are not ready to have sex at six weeks, and some women are ready before. Both you and your husband should understand that this is very individual.

Q *It's been two weeks since my delivery. Can I lift grocery sacks, or should I still avoid lifting?*

A During the first two weeks we recommend that you don't lift anything heavier than the baby. After that, you can slowly increase your lifting, but until six weeks, try to avoid anything heavier than fifteen pounds (the equivalent of two gallons of milk).

Q *I'm afraid I'm not producing enough milk for my baby. How can I tell?*

A The number-one question of new mothers who breast-feed is related to breast milk supply—"Is it enough?" Instances in which a mother cannot produce enough milk are rare. Since we can't see how much our baby is getting, there are a few indicators that she is being adequately nourished. If your baby is having six to eight wet diapers per day, and three or more stools per day (after the first twenty-four to forty-eight hours) she is probably getting plenty. Remember, just because she seems to be hungry often, that does not mean she is not getting enough. Breast milk is easily digestible, so it's normal for your baby to want to eat often.

Q *I have breast implants and I am breast-feeding. Is that okay?*

A Yes. Breast implants should have little or no effect on your ability to breast-feed your baby. They have not been shown to limit or damage milk supply. There have been reports of more problems with painful engorgement among lactating women with breast implants. Those women are advised to follow the same strategies to relieve engorgement symptoms as women without implants.

Q *It has been eight weeks since my son was born, and my skin looks terrible. My face looks dry and dull, and it keeps breaking out. Is there anything I can do?*

A Yes. Women often are disappointed with their skin's appearance after childbirth. Hormonal changes, fatigue, and stress can cause skin to appear dry, wrinkled, and dull, and can even cause skin breakouts or acne. Don't be discouraged. You can improve your skin. There are several new skin products on the market today which have been shown to provide excellent results—rejuvenating and reviving skin's youthful texture and glow, and eliminating acne problems. Many products make exaggerated claims, making it confusing to figure out which ones actually work and which don't. For more information about effectively enhancing your skin's appearance, refer to the following page.

(Advisory Board: George Cole, M.D.; Scott Bailey, M.D.; James Romine, M.D.; David Buckley, M.D.; David Duke, M.D.; James Beckman, Jr., M.D.; Allison Morris, R.N.P., Kim Moody, M.S., R.D.; Sandy Trexler, Ed. D.; and Mike Trexler, Ph. D.)

■ CONSULTATION SERVICES AND PRODUCTS

DR. SANDRA TREXLER AND/OR DR. MIKE TREXLER are available for speaking engagements, workshops, seminars, and personal consultations. Sandy and Mike speak on a variety of subjects. Here are some of the more popular topics:

- ■ Women's health issues
- ■ Self-esteem and image
- ■ Physical fitness and nutrition
- ■ Body Contouring
- ■ Lifelong health and wellness
- ■ Stress management
- ■ Conflict resolution

For more information on the Trexlers' consultation services or premium line of advanced skin-care products, call them at (800) 443-7549. For the products themselves, refer to:

- ■ Fruit acid wrinkle reduction system
- ■ Acne control system
- ■ Rejuvenating moisturizer
- ■ Anti-bacterial facial cleanser

APPENDIX
BODY CONTOURING

REFER TO
CHAPTER 14

I

BODY CONTOURING
BASIC PROGRAM—WEEK 1

DAY	TOTAL MINUTES	WALKING PACE STEPS/15 SECONDS	FAT-BURNING MINUTES	DATE COMPLETED
1	20	SLOW	0	
2	30	SLOW	10	
3	20	MODERATE	0	
4	30	MODERATE	10	
5	REST	REST		
6	30	SLOW	10	
7	30	MODERATE	10	

SLOW=20-24 STEPS/15 SECONDS
MODERATE=25-29 STEPS/15 SECONDS
BRISK=30-34 STEPS/15 SECONDS
FAST=35+ STEPS/15 SECONDS

40 TOTAL FBMS

DAILY FAT RECORD

Write down each food you eat that has fat in it. Look carefully over this list at the end of Day 7. Find foods you can reduce or eliminate.

Day 1

Day 2

Day 3

Day 4

Day 5

Day 6

Day 7

BODY CONTOURING
BASIC PROGRAM—WEEK 2

DAY	TOTAL MINUTES	WALKING PACE STEPS/15 SECONDS	FAT-BURNING MINUTES	DATE COMPLETED
1	20	MODERATE	0	
2	30	SLOW	10	
3	30	MODERATE	10	
4	30	MODERATE	10	
5	REST	REST		
6	45	MODERATE	25	
7	30	SLOW	10	

SLOW=20-24 STEPS/15 SECONDS
MODERATE=25-29 STEPS/15 SECONDS
BRISK=30-34 STEPS/15 SECONDS
FAST=35+ STEPS/15 SECONDS

65 TOTAL FBMS

DAILY FAT RECORD

Write down each food you eat that has fat in it. Look carefully over this list at the end of Day 7. Find foods you can reduce or eliminate.

Day 1

Day 2

Day 3

Day 4

Day 5

Day 6

Day 7

BODY CONTOURING
BASIC PROGRAM—WEEK 3

DAY	TOTAL MINUTES	WALKING PACE STEPS/15 SECONDS	FAT-BURNING MINUTES	DATE COMPLETED
1	30	MODERATE	10	
2	30	MODERATE	10	
3	45	SLOW	25	
4	20	BRISK	0	
5	REST	REST		
6	45	MODERATE	25	
7	30	SLOW	10	

SLOW=20-24 STEPS/15 SECONDS
MODERATE=25-29 STEPS/15 SECONDS
BRISK=30-34 STEPS/15 SECONDS
FAST=35+ STEPS/15 SECONDS

80 TOTAL FBMS

DAILY FAT RECORD

Write down each food you eat that has fat in it. Look carefully over this list at the end of Day 7. Find foods you can reduce or eliminate.

Day 1

Day 2

Day 3

Day 4

Day 5

Day 6

Day 7

BODY CONTOURING
BASIC PROGRAM—WEEK 4

DAY	TOTAL MINUTES	WALKING PACE STEPS/15 SECONDS	FAT-BURNING MINUTES	DATE COMPLETED
1	30	SLOW	10	
2	45	SLOW	25	
3	45	MODERATE	25	
4	30	BRISK	10	
5	REST	REST		
6	45	MODERATE	25	
7	30	SLOW	10	
			105 TOTAL FBMS	

SLOW=20-24 STEPS/15 SECONDS
MODERATE=25-29 STEPS/15 SECONDS
BRISK=30-34 STEPS/15 SECONDS
FAST=35+ STEPS/15 SECONDS

DAILY FAT RECORD

Write down each food you eat that has fat in it. Look carefully over this list at the end of Day 7. Find foods you can reduce or eliminate.

Day 1

Day 2

Day 3

Day 4

Day 5

Day 6

Day 7

BODY CONTOURING
BASIC PROGRAM—WEEK 5

DAY	TOTAL MINUTES	WALKING PACE STEPS/15 SECONDS	FAT-BURNING MINUTES	DATE COMPLETED
1	45	MODERATE	25	_____
2	30	BRISK	10	
3	45	MODERATE	25	_____
4	30	BRISK	10	
5	REST	REST		_____
6	45	BRISK	25	
7	45	MODERATE	25	_____
		SLOW=20-24 STEPS/15 SECONDS	120 TOTAL	
		MODERATE=25-29 STEPS/15 SECONDS	FBMS	
		BRISK=30-34 STEPS/15 SECONDS		
		FAST=35+ STEPS/15 SECONDS		

DAILY FAT RECORD

Write down each food you eat that has fat in it. Look carefully over this list at the end of Day 7. Find foods you can reduce or eliminate.

Day 1

Day 2

Day 3

Day 4

Day 5

Day 6

Day 7

BODY CONTOURING
BASIC PROGRAM—WEEK 6

DAY	TOTAL MINUTES	WALKING PACE STEPS/15 SECONDS	FAT-BURNING MINUTES	DATE COMPLETED
1	45	MODERATE	25	
2	45	BRISK	25	
3	45	MODERATE	25	
4	30	BRISK	10	
5	REST	REST		
6	60	MODERATE	40	
7	45	MODERATE	25	

SLOW=20-24 STEPS/15 SECONDS
MODERATE=25-29 STEPS/15 SECONDS
BRISK=30-34 STEPS/15 SECONDS
FAST=35+ STEPS/15 SECONDS

150 TOTAL FBMS

DAILY FAT RECORD

Write down each food you eat that has fat in it. Look carefully over this list at the end of Day 7. Find foods you can reduce or eliminate.

Day 1

Day 2

Day 3

Day 4

Day 5

Day 6

Day 7

BODY CONTOURING
ADVANCED PROGRAM—WEEK 7
ACCELERATED FAT LOSS AND MUSCLE TONING

DAY	TOTAL MINUTES	WALKING PACE	FAT-BURNING MINUTES	FAST PACE @ 30 MIN.	DATE COMPLETED
1	45	BRISK	25		_____
2	30	BRISK	10		_____
3	60	SLOW	40		
4	60	MODERATE	40	(2x2 MIN.)	_____
5	REST	REST			
6	60	MODERATE	40		_____
7	45	BRISK	25		_____

SLOW=20-24 STEPS/15 SECONDS
MODERATE=25-29 STEPS/15 SECONDS
BRISK=30-34 STEPS/15 SECONDS
FAST=35+ STEPS/15 SECONDS

180 TOTAL FBMS

BOOSTER EXERCISES
WEEK 7

DAY	EXERCISE	NUMBER OF REPETITIONS	NUMBER OF SETS
1, 3, 6	ABDOMINAL CRUNCHES	10	2
1, 3, 6	MODIFIED PUSH-UPS	5	1

Number of Repetitions—Slowly complete the prescribed number of repetitions without stopping. Breathe normally; do not strain or hold your breath. Exhale as your muscles begin to contract.

Number of Sets—When you have completed the prescribed number of repetitions, you have completed one set. Do 10 crunches, 5 push-ups, and then 10 more crunches.

DAILY FAT RECORD

Write down each food you eat that has fat in it. Look carefully over this list at the end of Day 7. Find foods you can reduce or eliminate.

Day 1

Day 2

Day 3

Day 4

Day 5

Day 6

Day 7

BODY CONTOURING
ADVANCED PROGRAM—WEEK 8
ACCELERATED FAT LOSS AND MUSCLE TONING

DAY	TOTAL MINUTES	WALKING PACE	FAT-BURNING MINUTES	FAST PACE @ 30 MIN.	DATE COMPLETED
1	60	MODERATE	40	(2x2 MIN.)	
2	45	MODERATE	25		
3	60	SLOW	40		
4	45	MODERATE	25	(2x2 MIN.)	
5	REST	REST			
6	60	MODERATE	40		
7	45	MODERATE	25		

195 TOTAL FBMS

SLOW=20-24 STEPS/15 SECONDS
MODERATE=25-29 STEPS/15 SECONDS
BRISK=30-34 STEPS/15 SECONDS
FAST=35+ STEPS/15 SECONDS

BOOSTER EXERCISES

WEEK 8

DAY	EXERCISE	NUMBER OF REPETITIONS	NUMBER OF SETS
2, 4, 7	ABDOMINAL CRUNCHES	15	2
2, 4, 7	MODIFIED PUSH-UPS	10	1

Number of Repetitions—Slowly complete the prescribed number of repetitions without stopping. Breathe normally; do not strain or hold your breath. Exhale as your muscles begin to contract.

Number of Sets—When you have completed the prescribed number of repetitions, you have completed one set. Do 15 crunches, 10 push-ups, and then 15 more crunches.

DAILY FAT RECORD

Write down each food you eat that has fat in it. Look carefully over this list at the end of Day 7. Find foods you can reduce or eliminate.

Day 1

Day 2

Day 3

Day 4

Day 5

Day 6

Day 7

Body Contouring
Advanced Program—Week 9
Accelerated Fat Loss and Muscle Toning

DAY	TOTAL MINUTES	WALKING PACE	FAT-BURNING MINUTES	FAST PACE @ 30 MIN.	DATE COMPLETED
1	45	BRISK	25		_____
2	60	MODERATE	40		_____
3	45	MODERATE	25	(2x2 MIN.)	_____
4	60	MODERATE	40		_____
5	REST	REST			_____
6	60	MODERATE	40	(3x2 MIN.)	_____
7	60	SLOW	40		_____

210 TOTAL FBMS

SLOW=20-24 STEPS/15 SECONDS
MODERATE=25-29 STEPS/15 SECONDS
BRISK=30-34 STEPS/15 SECONDS
FAST=35+ STEPS/15 SECONDS

BOOSTER EXERCISES

WEEK 9

DAY	EXERCISE	NUMBER OF REPETITIONS	NUMBER OF SETS
2, 4, 7	ABDOMINAL CRUNCHES	20	2
2, 4, 7	MODIFIED PUSH-UPS	10	2

Number of Repetitions—Slowly complete the prescribed number of repetitions without stopping. Breathe normally; do not strain or hold your breath. Exhale as your muscles begin to contract.

Number of Sets—When you have completed the prescribed number of repetitions, you have completed one set. Do 20 crunches, 10 push-ups. Rest one minute, then repeat.

DAILY FAT RECORD

Write down each food you eat that has fat in it. Look carefully over this list at the end of Day 7. Find foods you can reduce or eliminate.

Day 1

Day 2

Day 3

Day 4

Day 5

Day 6

Day 7

BODY CONTOURING
ADVANCED PROGRAM—WEEK 10
ACCELERATED FAT LOSS AND MUSCLE TONING

DAY	TOTAL MINUTES	WALKING PACE	FAT-BURNING MINUTES	FAST PACE @ 30 MIN.	DATE COMPLETED
1	30	BRISK	25		
2	75	MODERATE	55		
3	45	BRISK	25	(2x2 MIN.)	
4	60	SLOW	40		
5	REST	REST			
6	60	MODERATE	40	(3x2 MIN.)	
7	60	MODERATE	40		

SLOW=20-24 STEPS/15 SECONDS
MODERATE=25-29 STEPS/15 SECONDS
BRISK=30-34 STEPS/15 SECONDS
FAST=35+ STEPS/15 SECONDS

225 TOTAL FBMs

BOOSTER EXERCISES

WEEK 10

DAY	EXERCISE	NUMBER OF REPETITIONS	NUMBER OF SETS
1, 3, 4, 7	ABDOMINAL CRUNCHES	25	2
1, 3, 4, 7	MODIFIED PUSH-UPS	15	2

Number of Repetitions—Slowly complete the prescribed number of repetitions without stopping. Breathe normally; do not strain or hold your breath. Exhale as your muscles begin to contract.

Number of Sets—When you have completed the prescribed number of repetitions, you have completed one set. Do 25 crunches, then 15 push-ups. Rest one minute and repeat.

You are now doing Booster Exercises 4 days per week.

DAILY FAT RECORD

Write down each food you eat that has fat in it. Look carefully over this list at the end of Day 7. Find foods you can reduce or eliminate.

Day 1

Day 2

Day 3

Day 4

Day 5

Day 6

Day 7

BODY CONTOURING
ADVANCED PROGRAM—WEEK 11
ACCELERATED FAT LOSS AND MUSCLE TONING

DAY	TOTAL MINUTES	WALKING PACE	FAT-BURNING MINUTES	FAST PACE @ 30 MIN.	DATE COMPLETED
1	45	BRISK	25		
2	60	MODERATE	40	(2x2 MIN.)	
3	75	SLOW	55		
4	45	MODERATE	25		
5	REST	REST			
6	75	MODERATE	55		
7	60	MODERATE	40	(3x2 MIN.)	

240 TOTAL FBMS

SLOW=20-24 STEPS/15 SECONDS
MODERATE=25-29 STEPS/15 SECONDS
BRISK=30-34 STEPS/15 SECONDS
FAST=35+ STEPS/15 SECONDS

BOOSTER EXERCISES

WEEK 11

DAY	EXERCISE	NUMBER OF REPETITIONS	NUMBER OF SETS
1, 3, 4, 6	ABDOMINAL CRUNCHES	35	2
1, 3, 4, 6	MODIFIED PUSH-UPS	20	2

Number of Repetitions—Slowly complete the prescribed number of repetitions without stopping. Breathe normally; do not strain or hold your breath. Exhale as your muscles begin to contract.

Number of Sets—When you have completed the prescribed number of repetitions, you have completed one set. Do 35 crunches, then 25 push-ups. Rest one minute, then repeat.

DAILY FAT RECORD

Write down each food you eat that has fat in it. Look carefully over this list at the end of Day 7. Find foods you can reduce or eliminate.

Day 1

Day 2

Day 3

Day 4

Day 5

Day 6

Day 7

BODY CONTOURING
ADVANCED PROGRAM—WEEK 12
ACCELERATED FAT LOSS AND MUSCLE TONING

DAY	TOTAL MINUTES	WALKING PACE	FAT-BURNING MINUTES	FAST PACE @ 30 MIN.	DATE COMPLETED
1	30	MODERATE	10		
2	75	SLOW	55		
3	60	MODERATE	40		
4	75	MODERATE	55	(3x2 MIN.)	
5	REST	REST			
6	60	MODERATE	40		
7	60	MODERATE	40		

240 TOTAL FBMS

SLOW=20-24 STEPS/15 SECONDS
MODERATE=25-29 STEPS/15 SECONDS
BRISK=30-34 STEPS/15 SECONDS
FAST=35+ STEPS/15 SECONDS

BOOSTER EXERCISES

WEEK 12

DAY	EXERCISE	NUMBER OF REPETITIONS	NUMBER OF SETS
1, 3, 6, 7	ABDOMINAL CRUNCHES	50	2
1, 3, 6, 7	MODIFIED PUSH-UPS	25	2

Number of Repetitions—Slowly complete the prescribed number of repetitions without stopping. Breathe normally; do not strain or hold your breath. Exhale as your muscles begin to contract.

Number of Sets—When you have completed the prescribed number of repetitions, you have completed one set.

Congratulations, this is the last week of your scheduled program. When you complete Day 7, rest for two consecutive days. You should feel energized and lean. Keep up the good work. When you finish, choose any week in the advanced program to maintain your fat-burning benefits.

DAILY FAT RECORD

Day 1

Day 2

Day 3

Day 4

Day 5

Day 6

Day 7

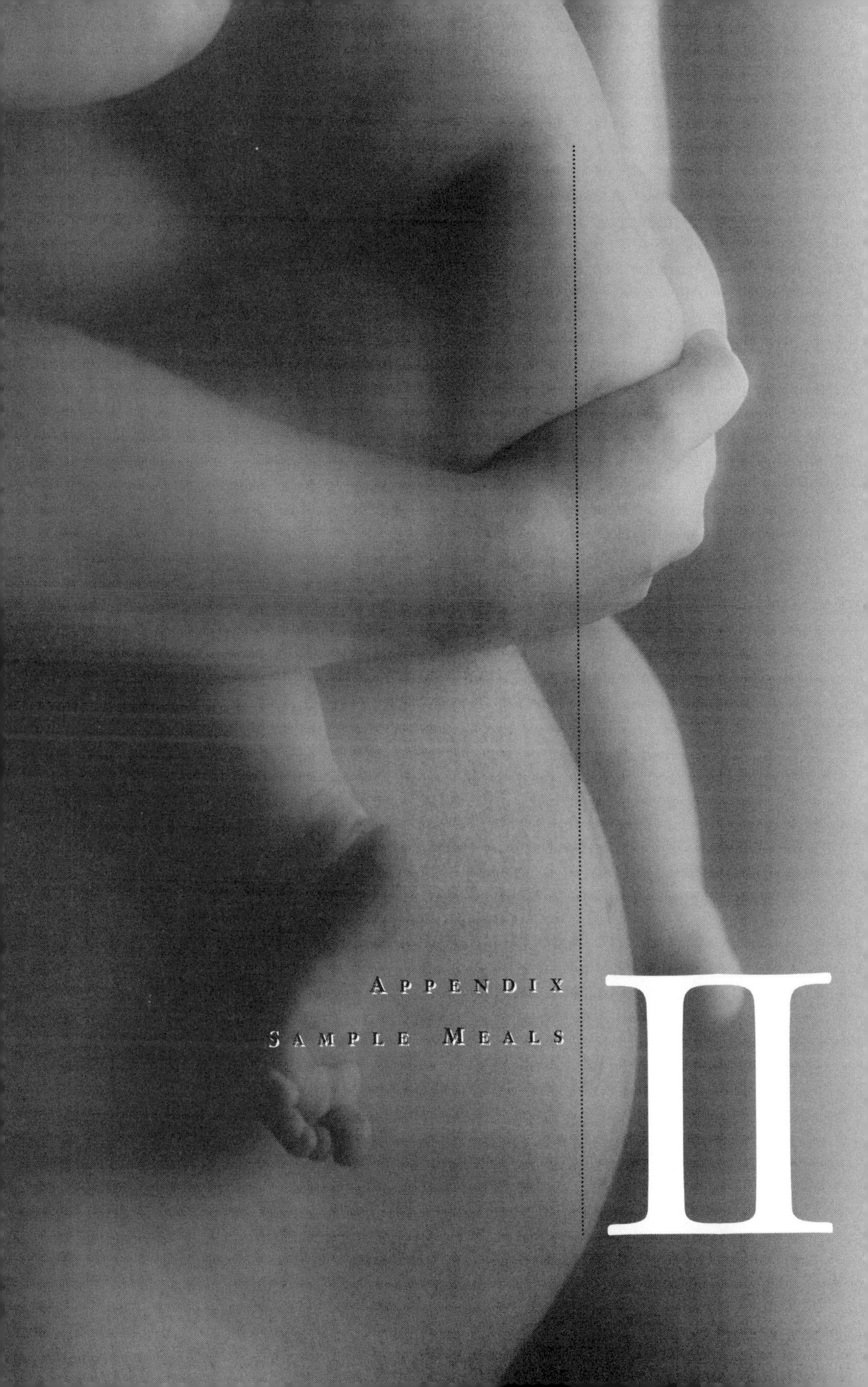

Appendix II

Sample Meals

*T*he following meals and snacks fit into the Body Contouring philosophy of eating. Each meal is designed to be prepared in fifteen minutes or less—since most new moms don't have a lot of extra time to spend in the kitchen. Many of the healthiest foods are those requiring the least amount of preparation. Less time in the kitchen means more time to devote to your walking program, and to other things you enjoy.

This is not a diet program intended for you to specifically follow. Rather, these are sample meals and snacks that promote health by reducing dietary fat. People often ask us during workshops—"What do you eat?" Here are the answers. This list includes many of the meals we eat on a regular basis.

Remember, diets don't work. You need to be able to eat the foods you like, to learn to prepare your foods in low-fat ways, and to gradually incorporate a greater variety of healthy, convenient, low-fat foods into your eating plan. We are not recommending that you eat exactly what we eat. We want you to become aware of the principles involved in low-fat, healthy eating, and use these principles in developing your eating philosophy.

SAMPLE BODY CONTOURING BREAKFASTS ■

ONE OF THE MAJOR COMPLAINTS I hear from women during the postpartum period is that they are constipated. The following recommendations should help keep you naturally regular.

Begin each morning with a large (ten-to-twelve-ounce) glass of water, followed by one of the following:

■ A small (six-ounce) glass of prune juice

■ An orange

■ A whole lemon squeezed into four ounces of water

After you've had your water and one of the items listed above, you can drink a cup of decaffeinated (or reduced-caffeine) coffee if you like. Then select a nutritious, high-fiber breakfast. An excellent choice would be:

Bowl of high-fiber cereal
Fiber One or All Bran
Skim milk
One piece of whole-wheat toast
Dry or topped with fat-free margarine and fruit spread

This breakfast is a good choice if you are having problems with constipation, because Fiber One and All Bran cereals contain about fourteen grams of dietary fiber as compared to Raisin Bran, which contains about four grams.

If constipation is not a problem, other healthy breakfast options include the following:

Bowl of medium-fiber cereal
Raisin Bran, Fruit and Fiber, Fruitful Bran
Skim milk
One piece of whole-wheat toast
Topped with fat-free margarine and fruit spread

Whole-wheat pancakes
Two four-inch diameter, prepared without oil
Fat-free margarine
Lite syrup
Large glass of skim milk

Low-fat or fat-free yogurt
Bagel with fat-free margarine and fruit spread

Low-fat or fat-free yogurt
Two pieces of raisin toast with fat-free margarine

Three pieces of whole-wheat toast
Topped with fat-free margarine and fruit spread
One medium banana
Glass of skim milk

Four egg whites scrambled
Two pieces whole-wheat toast
Topped with fat-free margarine and fruit spread
Glass of skim milk

Bowl of fresh fruit
One bagel
Topped with fat-free margarine and fruit spread, or two pieces of whole-wheat toast
Glass of skim milk

Three pieces of lite cinnamon toast
Prepared with fat-free margarine and lightly sprinkled with cinnamon and sugar or equal
Glass of skim milk

Two pieces of French toast
   Prepared by dipping wheat bread in mixture of egg white, skim milk, and cinnamon, and cooking it on dry skillet sprayed with cooking spray
Lite syrup or fruit spread
Glass of skim milk

English muffin
   Topped with fat-free margarine and fruit spread
Serving of fresh fruit
Glass of skim milk

Omelet
   Prepared with four egg whites, filled with fat-free cheese and salsa
Two pieces of whole-wheat toast with fat-free margarine
Skim milk

Cheese muffin
   Prepared by melting low-fat or fat-free cheese on an English muffin
Serving of fresh fruit
Glass of skim milk

Bran muffin
Serving of fresh or fresh frozen fruit
Glass of skim milk

One English muffin
Topped with turkey breast, two scrambled egg whites, and fat-free cheese (salsa, if you like)
Skim milk

SAMPLE BODY CONTOURING LUNCHES

Turkey breast sandwich on whole-wheat bread
Fat-free mayo or mustard, lettuce and tomato optional
Three to six low-fat or fat-free crackers
Harvest Grain, Snackwell, or other, or fat-free chips and salsa
Carrots and/or celery or other veggies

Tuna salad sandwich on whole-wheat bread
Prepare tuna with fat-free mayo, apples, celery, or other low-fat ingredients
Lettuce and tomato
Low-fat crackers
Carrots and cauliflower or broccoli
Dipped in fat-free ranch salad dressing

Chef salad
Prepared with assorted lettuce, raw veggies, turkey breast
Low-fat or nonfat cheese, and nonfat salad dressing
Low-fat crackers or piece of French bread

Pasta Salad
Cooked pasta tossed with fat-free Italian salad dressing, Parmesan cheese (could use fat-free) and Nature's Seasoning
Serving of raw veggies with fat-free dip
Crackers or toast (plain)

Baked potato
with Molly McButter, fat-free cheese, and/or nonfat Italian salad dressing, salsa
Serving of raw veggies

Fruit plate with nonfat yogurt
Crackers, toast, or raisin bread
Small serving of tuna or turkey breast

Fruit plate with nonfat cottage cheese
Crackers or toast
Small serving of turkey breast

SAMPLE BODY CONTOURING SUPPERS

Hamburgers
Made with diet lean ground beef. Cook and then drain all grease out of patties on paper towels. Serve with fat-free mayo, lettuce and tomato.
Baked potato fries
Bake potatoes, cut into small pieces, broil until crispy and serve like French fries.

Spaghetti and meat sauce
Prepare meat sauce by browning ground beef; drain and rinse all fat, then return to skillet and add onion, garlic, mushrooms, tomato sauce, etc.
Green salad with nonfat Italian dressing
French bread

Pasta with red sauce from a jar
Ragu's Today's Recipe, or other
Green salad with nonfat Italian dressing
Wheat rolls or other bread

Pasta with clam sauce
Cook pasta and season with Molly McButter and Nature's Seasoning. Add clams from the can with juice and stir. Top with Parmesan cheese.
Green salad or vegetable
French bread

Pasta salad
Cook pasta and add your choice of vegetables, which have been sautéed in chicken broth. Mix the veggies and the broth with the pasta and top with Parmesan cheese.
Green salad
French bread

Jumbo baked potatoes
Cook extra-large potatoes and top with sautéed vegetables and nonfat cheese.

French bread or low-fat wheat rolls
Green salad with nonfat Italian dressing

Chef salad
Prepared with assorted greens and topped with lean deli turkey or chicken and your choice of fresh vegetables and nonfat cheese

French or wheat bread
Rice-a-Roni
Prepared without butter—use chicken broth to brown

Baked chicken breast
Marinated in cooking wine, Worcestershire sauce, nonfat Italian dressing, etc.

Rice-a-Roni or baked potatoes
Prepared with defatted chicken broth instead of butter

Green salad or vegetable

Baked fish
Use lemon juice and Parmesan cheese.

Macaroni and cheese
Prepared from box with milk and no butter

Sautéed vegetables
Prepared in chicken broth

Boiled or grilled shrimp
Cocktail sauce
Baked potatoes
Green salad

Lean steak
Trim any fat, small portion
Mashed potatoes
Prepared with skim milk and spiced with Nature's Seasoning,
Molly McButter, or Butter Buds
Green salad

Fajitas
(Chicken or beef) sautéed in cooking wine or chicken broth.
Prepare meat in skillet with onions, green peppers, etc. Use whole
wheat or regular flour or corn tortillas, heated.
Lettuce and tomato
Nonfat cheese
Vegetarian refried beans
Salsa

Chicken Caesar Salad
Prepared with romaine lettuce, fat-free or low-fat mozzarella
cheese, and chicken cooked in a skillet in cooking wine and lemon
juice, topped with regular or fat-free Parmesan cheese
Serving of raw veggies
Sourdough or French bread with fat-free margarine

Low-fat pizza
Prepared using ready-made Boboli crust topped with sauce and a variety of veggies sautéed in fat-free chicken broth; fat-free or low-fat cheese; deli turkey or chicken
Small green salad

Soup
Healthy Choice from a can, or low-fat homemade
Deli turkey or chicken sandwich, or green salad with turkey
Nonfat chips or crackers and salsa

Low-fat chili
Prepared with 90-percent lean ground chuck or turkey breast. Brown meat, drain and rinse. Return to skillet and add chopped onion and garlic. Use one of the packaged chili mixes for seasoning, and add canned or fresh tomatoes and pinto beans.
Green salad

SAMPLE BODY CONTOURING SNACKS

SELECT THREE PER DAY, mid-morning, late-afternoon, and evening.

Piece of fresh fruit and nonfat yogurt

Frozen cherries or other fruit, and nonfat yogurt

Low-fat or nonfat yogurt and one graham cracker

One piece of toast with nonfat butter and fruit spread or low sugar jelly (eight calories per teaspoon)

Frozen or fresh fruit, and one serving of lite cool whip or fat-free cottage cheese

Canned pineapple chunks and serving of fat-free cottage cheese

Snackwell's fat-free or low-fat cookies (limit two per serving) and small glass of skim milk

Piece of raisin bread, plain or toasted (fat-free margarine and fruit spread optional)

Nonfat ice cream or frozen yogurt (could top with frozen fruit)

Low-fat or nonfat crackers, and nonfat cheese

Fat-free nachos (Top fat-free chips with fat-free cheese and broil until cheese is slightly melted—it might not melt completely the way fatty cheese does!)

Bagel topped with fat-free cream cheese

Glass of skim milk

Piece of toast with fruit spread or small amount of jelly

Fat-free snack cake (Hostess cupcake with one gram of fat) and small glass skim milk

Seventy-five percent reduced-fat popcorn with small glass skim milk

Nonfat saltine crackers or chips and salsa

Fat-free chips and salsa

Healthy Choice fat-free cheese sticks (one or two) and bagel or crackers

Nonfat or low-fat granola bar and small (six-ounce) glass of skim milk

Serving of raw veggies and fat-free dip, and small glass skim milk

Small (three-ounce) serving of tuna packed in water, or deli turkey or chicken, with crackers

Fat-free or low-fat bran muffin (or other) and small glass of skim milk

Fat-free, sugar-free hot chocolate, and one or two graham crackers

Small bowl of cereal and skim milk

Fat-free pretzels and skim milk

Dry cereal snack mix (mix two or three cereals you like together and keep in a container for a healthy snack) and a glass of skim milk

STRATEGIES FOR DEVELOPING YOUR INDIVIDUAL BODY CONTOURING EATING PHILOSOPHY

1 A *Body Contouring Eating Philosophy* encourages you to eat foods you like prepared in a low-fat way. Also eat smaller amounts, but more frequently throughout the day. Since you know you will be eating healthy snacks more often, you will be less likely to overeat at mealtime. You never have to go hungry with the *Body Contouring Plan,* so you never need to stuff yourself.

When you're eating a meal, tell yourself that you will be able to have a snack in an hour or so following that meal. That helps you remember that there is no need to overeat, and it gives you something to look forward to. It's a healthier way of eating, too, because by eating less volume at one time, we are less likely to convert excess calories into stored fat, and by eating more frequently, we are able to stimulate our metabolism many times throughout the day. Higher energy levels come with eating smaller amounts, more frequently.

2 Sometimes people experience hunger attacks. A hunger attack is a sudden feeling of extreme hunger that makes us feel like we must eat a large volume of food quickly. We advise our clients to take a short walk, clean house, or do some activity for ten minutes or so, and see if the hunger attack fades. If it doesn't, then go ahead and eat. Have healthy, low-fat foods available to satisfy the attack. These need to be foods you can eat in large quantities and foods which are bulky or filling.

Great foods for satisfying hunger attacks include:

SEVENTY-FIVE PERCENT REDUCED-FAT microwave popcorn (you can eat the whole bag if you need to, and only get three or four grams of fat—and plenty of volume), fat-free chips and salsa (you could eat half the bag and only get about three grams of fat—most salsa has no fat), or fat-free cereal. High-fiber cereals such as Fiber One work great for hunger attacks because they make us feel full and are very low in calories—eat these types of foods until you feel content!

3 Satisfy emotional hunger with something warm and smooth. What do we mean by emotional hunger? This is the type of hunger that is triggered when we feel sad or blue, or when we just need to be comforted. Maybe you had an argument with your husband or your mother, or the baby cried all night. The ideal snack for emotional hunger is fat-free, sugar-free hot chocolate. You can prepare it in the microwave in minutes and sip it for a long time. Nursing this chocolate, creamy treat makes us feel warm and cozy—and it only has fifty calories (no fat) and is a good source of calcium. If you still aren't satisfied, have another cup.

4 Give in to a strong craving for a chocolate fix with a rich chocolate flavor, low-fat snack. A delicious way to satisfy your chocolate tooth is to eat Hostess Light Chocolate Cupcakes with creamy filling. They have 70 percent less fat than regular cupcakes, with only one gram of fat and 120 calories per cupcake. You could even eat two, and still not stray from your eating philosophy—yet thoroughly satisfy your craving for chocolate. Other options include Snackwell's chocolate fudge cookies, or fat-free chocolate ice cream.

5 Avoid nibbling away at your toddler's high-fat foods. For example, if you make her a peanut butter and jelly sandwich, it is very tempting to nibble or eat the portion she leaves behind. Instead, prepare a low-fat snack for yourself to eat while you feed her. When she is done, wrap up the remainder of her sandwich or snack immediately, and give it to her later, or throw it away. Break the habit of unconscious nibbling at your children's food. Remember, she needs the fat, but you don't.

6 Drink a large glass of water before you eat a meal or snack. Often, we mistake signals of thirst for hunger. If you think you're getting hungry, drink first. You may only be thirsty. Even if you're still hungry, you'll likely eat less after drinking a large glass of water.

7 Develop the habit of evaluating everything that could potentially go into your mouth. We told you not to avoid foods you love. But we still want you to go through the process of evaluating them before you eat them. For example, is that package of M & M's worth the fourteen grams of fat which will likely be deposited in your fat cells, or would you be just as satisfied with a Hostess cupcake which yields only one gram of fat? If, after evaluating the benefit versus the cost of eating a fattening food, you still desire to eat it—then go ahead.

We like to talk about foods in terms of benefit versus cost. What do we mean? Fattening foods offer the benefit of tickling your taste buds for a few seconds, but the cost is that they load themselves into your fat cells, making you larger. Healthy foods might offer less immediate appeal to the taste buds (this is the only cost), but offer the major benefit of enhancing your body's health, performance, and appearance.

So we learn to think of food in terms of benefit/cost. Remember, if you do eat a fattening food, keep each bite in your mouth as long as you can, because the only benefit it offers is the few seconds of pleasure it brings your taste buds. Don't feel guilty when you eat it, because you evaluated the benefit/cost and you made a choice—and that's a good sign. Since these types of indulgences take you away from your Body Contouring goals, we believe in time you will learn to desire lower-fat alternatives.

8 Avoid eating what we call "hungry foods" in private. These are foods we eat which trigger something inside us that makes us lose control. We want more and more. They are usually fattening foods which have no tangible beginning and end point—so we have no limits. Examples of hungry foods are ice cream, pizza, candies such as M&M's, bite-size chocolates, etc., nuts of all kinds, donuts and pastries, breakfast meats such as bacon or sausage, scrambled eggs, peanut butter, regular chips and salsa, French fries, and fattening deserts such as cobblers, pies, cookies, and cakes.

Many times we will avoid eating, for example, a small piece of cake with everyone else at our child's birthday party. But when everyone leaves, we take a small bite off the remaining cake. That bite triggers our hungry alarm and before we know it, we've eaten the rest of the cake. Instead of making this mistake, eat hungry foods only in the presence of others, and set and stick to limits. That means cut a reasonably sized piece of cake and eat it with everyone else. Let someone else take the leftovers home. If you've identified substitutes you find just as satisfying, such as low-fat cupcakes, eat your low-fat dessert while everyone else loads their fat cells.

9 Since we want low-fat meals to become a way of life, learn to prepare your favorite foods in a low-fat way, and learn new low-fat options. The following are some tips for low-fat food preparation:

- Use nonfat cooking sprays, cooking wine, lemon juice, or defatted chicken broth instead of oil to sauté or pan-fry foods.

- Omit oil from recipes, and substitute another liquid, such as apple sauce or Karo syrup.

- Avoid using whole eggs. If recipes call for one egg, use two egg whites or egg substitutes.

■ Trim all visible fat from meats, and remove skin before cooking.

■ Drain, then rinse ground meat after cooking to remove excess fat.

■ Use skim or fat-free dairy products.

RESOURCES

Auvenshire, M.A., and Enriquez, M.G. *Comprehensive Maternity Nursing: Perinatal and Women's Health.* 2d ed. Boston, Massachusetts: Jones and Bartlett, 1990.

Blair, Steven, P.E.D.; Clark, Debra G., M.S.; Cooper, Kenneth, M.D., M.P.H.; Gibbons, Larry W., M.D., M.P.H.; Kohl, Harold W. III, M.S.P.H.; and Paffenberger, Ralph F. Jr., M.D., Ph. D. "Physical Fitness and All-Cause Mortality: A Prospective Study of Healthy Men and Women." *Journal of the American Medical Association.* Chicago, Illinois: American Medical Association, November 3, 1989.

Dewey, Kathryn G., Ph.D.; Lonnerdal, Bo, Ph.D.; Lovelady, Cheryl A., Ph.D.; McCrory, Megan A., M.S.; and Nommsen-Rivers, Laurie A., M.S. "A Randomized Study of the Effects of Aerobic Exercise by Lactating Women on Breast-Milk Volume and Composition." *The New England Journal of Medicine.* Massachusetts Medical Society, February 17, 1994.

Eisenberg, Arlene. *What to Expect the First Year.* New York: Workman, 1989.

Ellis, Albert and Harper, Robert. *A Guide to Rational Living.* Englewood Cliffs, New Jersey: Prentice-Hall, 1961.

Food and Nutrition Board, Institute of Medicine, National Academy of Sciences. *Nutrition During Pregnancy and Lactation: An Implementation Guide.* Washington, D.C.: National Academy Press, 1992.

Freedman, R. Bodylove. *Learning to Like Our Looks and Ourselves.* New York: Harper and Row, 1988.

Gant, Norman F., MacDonald, Paul C., and Pritchard, Jack A. *Williams Obstetrics.* 17th ed. East Norwalk, Connecticut: Appleton-Century-Crofts, 1985.

Hahn, Dale and Payne, Wayne A. *Understanding Your Health*. St. Louis, Missouri: Mosby Year Book, 1992.

Harley, Willard F., Jr. *His Needs, Her Needs: Building an Affair-Proof Marriage*. Tarrytown, New York: The Fleming H. Revell Company, 1986.

Johnson,Caesar. *To See a World in a Grain of Sand*. C.R. Gibson Company: Norwalk, Connecticut, 1972.

Katch, Frank I., Katch, Victor L., and McArdle, William D. *Exercise Physiology*. 3rd ed. Philadelphia/London: Lea and Febiger, 1991.

Mercer, R. "The Nurse and Maternal Tasks of Early Postpartum." *The American Journal of Maternal Child Nursing*. New York: The American Journal of Nursing Company, September-October 1981.

Naeye, R. "Weight Gain and the Outcome of Pregnancy." *American Journal of Obstetrics and Gynecology*. St. Louis, Missouri: Mosby Year Book, 1979.

Winston, S. *Getting Organized*. New York, New York: Warner Books, 1978.

I N D E X